W9-BFY-061

ALSO BY LAWRENCE L. WEED

Medical Records, Medical Education and Patient Care

Your Health Care and How To Manage It

Knowledge Coupling: New Premises and New Tools for Medical Care and Education

MEDICINE IN DENIAL

Published Version 1.02, February 2013
Available for purchase at www.createspace.com/3508751

Look for future information at www.world3medicine.com
(site to be constructed)

Printed in the United States of America
Printed by Createspace

ISBN: 1456417061
ISBN-13: 9781456417062

MEDICINE IN DENIAL

Lawrence L. Weed and Lincoln Weed

To the memory of Laura Brooks Weed

Contents

Overview x

I.   Introduction: Building a New System 1

II. Disorder and Denial in Medical Practice 15
     A. Failure in medical decision making—a case study 15
         1. Missing an obvious diagnosis 15
         2. How it happened 16
            a. Summary of the case 17
            b. The article's analysis 20
            c. A different analysis 22
            d. Further analyses from readers 25
     B. Implications for reform of medical practice 28
         1. Medicine's division of intellectual labor 28
         2. Implications of changing medicine's division of labor 31
            a. The significance of information technology 31
            b. The nature of disorder in medical decision making 33
            c. Basic implications for health care reform 36
            d. Consumer-driven spending and consumer-driven care 39

III. The Concept of Defined Inputs 43
     A. The need for defined inputs 43
     B. Modes of defining inputs 46
     C. Failings of "evidence-based medicine" as a mode of control
         over cognitive inputs 51

IV. The Foundation: Coupling Patient Data With Medical Knowledge 53
     A. Defining initial inputs as the foundation of care 53
     B. The structure of the initial workup 56
     C. Two contrasting approaches to the initial workup 58
     D. The basis for choosing between the two approaches 61
     E. Objections to the combinatorial approach 67
     F. A software implementation of the combinatorial approach 69
     G. Answering objections to the combinatorial approach 80

1. Feasibility of detailed initial data collection.................................80
2. Utility of detailed initial data 85
3. Utility of standardized initial data 89
4. Effect on the doctor-patient relationship.................................92
5. Information processing, clinical judgment and the two stages of decision making...97
   a. Analysis as information processing 97
   b. The two stages of decision making and the proper role of judgment 99
   c. Physician objections to separate stages of decision making ... 100

V. **"Idols of the Mind": Medicine, Science, and Commerce 105**
  A. Medicine and the development of science 105
   1. Intellect and the culture of science 106
   2. Intellect and the culture of medicine...............................111
    a. Alternative concepts of expertise 112
    b. Comparing scientific research and medical practice..........117
  B. Economy of knowledge in decision making 120
   1. The domain of commerce..120
   2. Comparing commerce and medicine...................................123
   3. The need for simple rules to manage complex information....126

VI. **Building on the Foundation: The Medical Record 131**
  A. The nature of complex cases 131
  B. The role of the medical record in bringing order and transparency to complex cases.......................................133
  C. The medical record and the four phases of medical action 145
   1. The database 145
   2. The problem list..152
    a. Defining medical problems 153
    b. Scope of the problem list.......................................155
   3. Initial plans..159
   4. Progress notes 166
  D. Further perspectives on the POMR..169
   1. Criticisms of the POMR...169
   2. The POMR and its integration with knowledge coupling from an IT perspective 171
   3. Resistance to the POMR...173

VII. The Gap Between Medical Knowledge and Individual Patients **177**

    A.   General knowledge and the individual patient 179

        1. Two forms of medical knowledge 179

            a. Population-based knowledge........................... 179

            b. Knowledge about individual variation 180

        2. The concept of individual uniqueness 181

    B.   Some implications 182

        1. The gap between evidence-based medicine and individual patient needs 182

        2. Medical practice and research 189

VIII. Medical Education and Credentialing as Barriers to Progress **195**

    A.   Extending the health care reform agenda to medical education and credentialing.. 195

        1. A century of stagnation 195

        2. The medical school experience 197

        3. Changing medical education from a knowledge-based to a skills-based approach 204

    B.   Marketplace implications of skills-based credentialing.................. 210

        1. Professional autonomy and regulation of practitioners............ 210

        2. Transforming the hierarchy of practitioners 212

IX. Education and the Role of the Patient/Consumer.................................... **221**

    A.   Autonomy.. 221

    B.   Education 228

APPENDIX A Analysis of two clinical trials................................ 235

APPENDIX B Scientific principles that tell us why people must manage their own health care.. 253

Authors' Background and Acknowledgements **267**

Overview

Essential to health care reform are two elements: standards of care for managing clinical information (analogous to accounting standards for managing financial information), and electronic tools designed to implement those standards. Both elements are external to the physician's mind. Although in large part already developed, these elements are virtually absent from health care. Without these elements, the physician continues to be relied upon as a repository of knowledge and a vehicle for information processing. The resulting disorder blocks health information technology from realizing its enormous potential, and deprives health care reform of an essential foundation. In contrast, standards and tools designed to integrate detailed patient data with comprehensive medical knowledge make it possible to define the data and knowledge taken into account for decision making. Similarly, standards for organizing patient data over time in medical records make it possible to trace connections among the data collected, the patient's problems, the practitioner's assessments, the actions taken, the patient's progress, the patient's behaviors and ultimate outcomes.

Two basic standards of care, and corresponding tools, bring order and transparency to medical decision making:

- First, from the outset of care, relevant patient data must be chosen, and its implications determined, based on the best available medical knowledge, independent of the limited personal knowledge of the practitioners involved. Patient data must be systematically linked to medical knowledge in a combinatorial manner, *before* the exercise of clinical judgment, using information tools to elicit all possibilities relevant to the problem situation, while defining and documenting the information taken into account. Practitioners' clinical judgments may add to, but must not subtract from, high standards of accuracy, completeness and objectivity for that information.

- Second, in complex cases, particularly in cases of chronic disease, the organization of data in medical records must be optimized for managing multiple problems over time. This means that each medical record must begin with a complete list of carefully defined patient problems, and that other clinical information in the record must be linked to the problem or problems to which it relates. Without that structure for the medical record, decisions are made out of context, follow-up and coordination of care are haphazard, and records are not usable for rigorous clinical research.

With these two basic standards of care, and the information tools needed to implement them, practitioners and patients can manage the flood of detailed information required for sound decision making over time. With this detailed information, made usable for research in structured electronic medical records, medical care can become increasingly refined and individualized. In contrast, so-called "evidence-based medicine" is derived from large population studies that fail to account for the medical uniqueness of each patient.

Enforcing the necessary standards and tools depends on changing medicine's culture of professional autonomy for highly educated physicians. Indeed, the concept of a physician as we know it is not viable. All practitioners must submit to meticulous definition and control of their inputs to care (a principle recognized by the patient safety movement). The primary barrier to this cultural change is graduate medical education and credentialing. These social institutions (1) fail to define, disseminate and enforce high standards of quality for provider inputs to care, (2) inhibit effective design and use of information technology to manage clinical information, and (3) suppress competition among providers who might otherwise exploit information technology to generate remarkable advances in patient care and medical knowledge.

I.
Introduction:
Building a New System

It is in vain to expect any great progress in the sciences by the superinducing or engrafting new matters upon old. An instauration must be made from the very foundations, if we do not wish to revolve forever in a circle, making only some slight and contemptible progress.

— *Francis Bacon*[1]

A culture of denial subverts the health care system from its foundation. The foundation—the basis for deciding what care each patient individually needs—is connecting patient data to medical knowledge. That foundation, and the processes of care resting upon it, are built by the fallible minds of physicians. A new, secure foundation requires two elements external to the mind: electronic information tools and standards of care for managing clinical information.

Electronic information tools are now widely discussed, but the tools depend on standards of care that are still widely ignored. The necessary standards for managing clinical information are analogous to accounting standards for managing financial information. If businesses were permitted to operate without accounting standards, the entire economy would be crippled. That is the condition in which the $2½ trillion U.S. health care system finds itself—crippled by lack of standards of care for managing clinical information. The system persists in a state of denial about the disorder that our own minds create, and that the missing standards of care would expose.

This pervasive disorder begins at the system's foundation. Contrary to what the public is asked to believe, physicians are not educated to connect patient data with medical knowledge safely and effectively. Rather than building that

---

1 Bacon F. *Novum Organon* (1620), Summary of the Second Part, Aphorisms Concerning the Interpretation of Nature and the Kingdom of Man, Aphorism No. 31 (Montague, trans., 1854); at http://history.hanover.edu/texts/Bacon/APHOR.html.

secure foundation for decisions, physicians are educated to do the opposite—to rely on personal knowledge and judgment—in denial of the need for external standards and tools. Medical decision making thus lacks the order, transparency and power that enforcing external standards and tools would bring about.

A simple example will illustrate medicine's missing foundation. Consider a person with chest pain. Careful review of the literature shows that a practitioner investigating this symptom needs to take into account approximately 100 diagnostic possibilities, involving most medical specialties. Each diagnostic possibility is definable as a combination of simple, inexpensive findings from the history, physical and basic laboratory tests. Checking all of the findings for all of the diagnostic possibilities results in approximately 440 findings on each patient. Each positive finding suggests one or more of the diagnostic possibilities. Each patient's particular combination of positive findings can be matched against all of the combinations of findings representing the diagnostic possibilities for chest pain. The output of this matching process is an *individualized* set of diagnostic possibilities, plus the patient's positive and negative findings for each. These findings constitute initial evidence for and against each possibility. The total set of possibilities (i.e. those for which at least one positive finding is made) represents the diagnoses worth considering for that patient. External tools generate this output by simple matching, without dependence on the fallible minds of costly physicians. The tools distill this output from the accumulated experience of countless patients and practitioners—experience that would be otherwise lost.

This meticulous matching process is feasible only with software tools. The minds of physicians do not have command of all the medical knowledge involved. Nor do physicians have the time to carry out the intricate matching of hundreds of findings on the patient with all the medical knowledge relevant to interpreting those findings. External tools are thus essential. But the tools are trustworthy only when their design and use conform to rigorous standards of care for managing clinical information.

Without the necessary standards and tools, the matching process is fatally compromised. Physicians resort to a shortcut process of highly educated guesswork. They begin with guesses about diagnostic possibilities that might account for the chest pain. Sometimes very sophisticated, these initial guesses lead to further guesswork about what to check during the initial history, physical examination and laboratory tests for investigating whatever diagnostic possibilities come to mind. And then physicians make more guesses about what the data mean, which in turn shapes their judgments about what further data to collect. Varying from one physician to another, these highly educated guesses are not explicit—

physicians do not carefully record their thinking or the information they take into account. Inputs to decision making are thus undefined.

We use the term "guesses" because these key initial judgments are made on the fly, *during* the patient encounter, based on whatever enters the physician's mind at the time. That mind may be highly informed and intelligent, but inevitably its judgments reflect limited personal knowledge and experience, and limited time for thought. Euphemistically termed "clinical judgment," physician thought processes cause a fatal voltage drop in transmitting complex knowledge and applying it to patient data. The outcome is that the entire health care enterprise lacks a secure foundation.

Equally insecure are the complex processes built on that foundation: decision making, execution, feedback and corrective action over time. Responsibility for all these processes falls on the mind of the physician. Here again the mind lacks external tools and accounting standards for managing clinical information.

Medical practice is thus trapped in a subjective realm. Unlike scientific practitioners, medical practitioners do not operate in an objective realm, where the *contents* of thought and knowledge exist independently of the individual mind, a realm where knowledge can be reliably transmitted and applied, where new knowledge can be rapidly translated into practice, where all knowledge can be tested against patient realities. Isolated from this objective realm, the mind becomes a negative force, a cause of confusion and disorder. Physicians are not equipped to fulfill their immense responsibility safely and effectively. Other practitioners are not equipped to share that responsibility with physicians. Patients are not equipped to work effectively with multiple practitioners, nor to assume the ultimate burden of decision making over their own bodies and minds. Third parties are not equipped to create order out of this chaos. Practitioners and patients are not accountable for their own behaviors, while third parties are left free to manipulate disorder for their own advantage.

In short, essential standards of care, information tools and feedback mechanisms are missing from the marketplace. These missing elements are in large part already developed (see parts IV and VI below). Yet, the underlying medical culture does not even recognize their absence. This does not prevent some practitioners from becoming virtuoso performers in narrow specialties or skills. But their virtuosity is personal, not systemic, and limited, not comprehensive. Missing is a total system for enforcing high quality care by all practitioners for all patients.

Medical school fills this vacuum with harmful habits and illusions that physicians find difficult to let go. Credentialing then confers a legal monopoly on physicians, insulating them from competition and preserving their illusions. The resulting state of denial blocks development of a secure, orderly, integrated system of defined inputs, tight feedback, clear accountability, and continuous improvement in patient care.

A system of that kind (see the diagram at the end of this Introduction) is the subject of this book. At first glance, this subject matter may seem like just a variation on current policy concerns with using "health information technology" to bring "evidence-based medicine" to "patient-centered" care. Yet, current policy fails to comprehend the needed discipline in medical practice and thus fails to define precisely what is needed from health information technology. A dangerous paradox thus exists: the power of technology to access information without limits magnifies the very problem of information overload that the technology is expected to solve. Solving that problem demands a meticulous, highly organized, explicit process of initial information processing, followed by careful problem definition, planning, execution, feedback, and corrective action over time, all documented under strict medical accounting standards. When this rigor is enforced, a promising paradox occurs: clarity emerges from complexity.

No such relief from complexity is in sight now. A wide gap exists between current reform initiatives and the disciplined medical practice that patients need. This gap exists regardless of whether health care is public or private, and regardless of whether health care spending is provider-driven (traditional fee-for-service medicine), payer-driven (managed care) or now "consumer-driven." Until the gap is closed, attempts at cost control and quality improvement will continue to revolve in a circle, without sustainable progress.

In contrast, were we to close the gap between medical practice and patient needs, society then could find enormous opportunities to harvest resources now going to waste. These wasted resources include not only vast sums spent on low-value care but also a vast body of medical knowledge that all patients and practitioners could use more effectively, simple tests and observations that in combination could uncover solutions to patient problems, patients who could become better equipped and motivated to improve their own health behaviors, routine patient care that could become a fertile source of new medical knowledge, and the firsthand insights of practitioners and patients who could participate in harvesting that new knowledge for their own benefit.

Closing the gap between medical practice and patient needs would transform how medicine is personally experienced by practitioners and patients alike.

Practitioners could find their work to be less exhausting and more rewarding, emotionally and intellectually, than what they now undergo. The physician's role could disaggregate into multiple roles, all freed from the impossible burdens of performance that physicians are now expected to bear. The expertise of nurses and other non-physician practitioners could deepen, and their roles could be elevated. All practitioners could follow time-honored standards of care that in the past have been honored more in the breach than the observance. All practitioners and patients could jointly use electronic information tools for matching data with medical knowledge, radically expanding their capacity to cope with complexity. All could use structured medical records, whose structure would itself bring order and transparency to the complex processes of care. Inputs by practitioners could thus be defined and subjected to constant feedback and improvement. A truly evidence-based medicine could develop, where evidence would be used to individualize care rather than standardize it. And a system of checks and balances could develop, where patients and practitioners would act on incentives for quality and economy far more effectively than before.

Were such a transformation to occur, each patient/consumer could engage in health care as a personal pursuit, navigating the health care delivery system as a transparent network for that purpose. Compare the transportation system—like health care, a system where public safety is at stake. Travelers rely on expert service providers when needed (pilots, auto mechanics, travel agents, for example), but the primary decision makers are travelers themselves. They determine the destination, the route, and the mode of travel for a journey. And their decisions are highly individualized. Two different people driving across the country might choose completely different routes, depending on whom and what they wish to visit and what they encounter along the way. Because such factors are variable, the choice of routes among different travelers is variable. No one would regard such variation as inappropriate. No one would expect travelers to conform to some "evidence-based" determination by experts of the "best" route across the country. Similarly, in medicine, no one should think that two different people labeled with the "same" disease necessarily have comparable medical needs. No one should think that the care of unique individuals must conform to "evidence-based" guidelines derived from "comparative effectiveness research" on large population databases. Effectiveness is context-specific. High quality, efficient care would thus emerge case-by-case, each person finding a different pathway in a progression of many small steps, with each step carefully chosen, reliably executed and accurately documented. Researchers could then study and correct any difficulties at each step, thereby assuring a better outcome for those who use that step in reaching their goal. This would mean continuous, incremental improvements throughout the medical landscape.

Like the transportation system, the health care system should be usable by ordinary consumers when feasible. In travel, rather than relying on taxi drivers, we learn to drive and we buy our own cars. Instead of hiring engineers to tell us what cars to buy, we read *Consumer Reports* and judge our personal needs and preferences for ourselves. Rather than hiring guides, we read maps and road signs, choosing routes for ourselves. Coming and going in all directions, we collectively shape the system with our choices. Experts and regulators then obtain feedback for system improvements.

In some modes of travel (rail and air), we depend on expert service providers, but we as consumers, not those experts, choose the mode of travel. By comparison, if transportation were like health care, then experts in the costliest mode of travel would monopolize authority to choose and the entire system would be distorted: pilots would decide when consumers travel by air, unnecessary flights for short distances would be routine, unnecessary airports would be built, the infrastructure for other modes of travel would be underdeveloped, and the choices available to consumers would be restricted.

Consumers in the transportation system depend on reliability of the infrastructure and transparency in the rules for its use. Consider auto transportation. Roads and bridges are maintained in drivable condition. Maps, road signs and electronic systems are provided for navigation. Drivers are licensed and cars inspected. Traffic laws are defined and enforced. Traffic patterns are monitored, safety threats are identified and each element of the infrastructure is improved as needed. Statistical information is used to inform these improvement efforts, not to prescribe "evidence-based" routes that travelers must follow. As a result, drivers can choose their routes, find their destinations and arrive safely. The primary risk to safety is the behaviors of other drivers, not breakdowns in the transportation system. In contrast, breakdowns in the safety, quality and economy of health care are epidemic.

Consider also airline safety regulation. It carefully defines inputs by workers with specialized expertise, and they function within an integrated system, every component of which is subject to strict scrutiny and control. Airline mechanics, for example, are subject to strict recordkeeping and inspection requirements. Pilot credentials are based not on formal education but on periodic demonstration of actual competence in flying specific classes of plane. Air traffic control systems, sophisticated cockpit instrumentation and detailed standards of care govern the actions of expert pilots. Pilots do not have professional autonomy.

They function within a protective system that is meticulously monitored. As a result, airline travel is so safe that no one chooses among airlines by comparing crash rates or pilot credentials.

Our description of the transportation system is, of course, oversimplified and idealized. But this underlines our point. Even with its failings, the transportation system is still far superior to the health care system in the quality of its parts and their connections.

In any complex system, all parts must be reliable and oriented towards a common general purpose, a purpose that different individuals specify and pursue in their own ways. The connections must generate corrective feedback loops, so that individual and collective actions remain compatible with the common general purpose.

In medicine that purpose is individualized medical problem solving. For that purpose, the health care system will never be trustworthy or affordable until its parts and their connections are reformed in three key respects. Indeed, health care's recent evolution is turning in these directions:

- *Inputs by practitioners must be carefully defined and controlled.* During the last 15 years, this development has begun to take root. The patient safety movement has demonstrated over and over again the need to define and control inputs from fallible human beings. But this development has focused largely on execution of decisions. Decision making itself equally needs definition and control of inputs from the human mind. Left to its own devices, the mind is unreliable and not well connected to other system components on which its inputs depend. Medical education and credentialing block the necessary changes in this regard. To bring inputs under control, the legal monopoly of physicians over medical practice must end, while medical education and credentialing for all practitioners must focus on instilling a core of behavior, not a core of knowledge. That means licenses to practice must be based on actual performance under standards of care defined by the system, not on learning fragments of the vast knowledge built into the system.

- *A trustworthy and transparent intellectual infrastructure for care must be established.* During the last 15 years, the Internet has revolutionized access to expanding medical knowledge. But the human mind cannot apply complex knowledge effectively without external aids. Practitioners and patients trying to navigate the medical landscape need two information tools: a map of the landscape and a communication system for the journey (see parts IV and VI below, respectively). The map (tools for coupling medical knowledge with patient-specific data) reveals the landscape so that individuals can find routes fitting their personal needs (unlike "evidence-based" travel directions dictated in advance). The communication system (structured medical records) enables the patient and multiple practitioners to coordinate their actions, planning and recording each step of the journey, informed by continuous feedback. With this infrastructure, all practitioners and consumers can apply complex knowledge to detailed data, and readily understand how their efforts interrelate.

- *The central role of the patient/consumer must be recognized.* During the last decade, this recognition has become increasingly evident in two areas: consumer-driven health care and management of chronic illness. But these developments are incomplete. The consumer-driven care movement focuses more on spending than care. In management of chronic illness, many organizations have developed approaches for helping patients manage their own conditions, but these disparate efforts are not unified by common tools and standards applicable in all medical contexts. The missing tools and standards exploit basic principles of orderly problem-solving that everyone grasps. With that simplicity and unity, the health system becomes transparent and usable for all.

We need to see health care not as an esoteric domain for specialized experts but as a universal human pursuit. To enable that pursuit, the culture of medicine and its intellectual infrastructure must both be transformed, reoriented towards individualized medical problem solving by and for each unique patient. That orientation differs fundamentally from evidence-based medicine, payer-driven managed care and traditional, provider-driven medicine. These are all variations on the same vendor-driven non-system of care. These variations are disconnected from patient needs because a truly consumer-driven system of care has yet to be built.

To present these concepts, we begin with a detailed case study (part II.A). Then we analyze some of its implications (parts II.B and III). Next, we describe two information tools[2], the standards of care they implement (parts IV and VI)

---

2 Specifically, the information tools are (1) decision support software designed for coupling medical knowledge with patient data, and (2) electronic medical records designed to organize care around patient problems instead of provider habits. Known respectively as knowledge coupling software and the problem-oriented medical record (POMR), these tools implement standards of care for managing medical information, as discussed in parts IV and VI below. Some basic references are Weed, LL., et al., *Knowledge Coupling: New Premises and New Tools for Medical Care Education*, New York: Springer-Verlag, 1991 (see especially chapter 13 of this volume,

and their relationship to the domains of science and commerce (part V). Finally, we analyze implications for the development of medical knowledge, medical education, and the patient's role (parts VII, VIII and IX, respectively). The diagram following this Introduction shows the basic elements of a total system of care. Appendix A analyzes two clinical trials of the software tools discussed in part IV. Appendix B further analyzes the patient's role.

All readers should begin with the case study in part II.A, which later sections reference repeatedly. After the case study, readers whose most immediate interests are the standards and tools for clinicians may wish to proceed directly to parts IV and VI. Other readers may wish to read each part sequentially. Regardless, each part is best understood in light of all the others. Reading the entire book is essential to fully understanding its core ideas. The following outline of Parts II to IX should further help orient the reader.

II   *Disorder in medical practice.* This part begins with a detailed case study of a missed diagnosis, showing why accepted practices inevitably produce such cases. Then we analyze some basic implications for reform of medical practice. The central concept is that medicine needs a new division of intellectual labor. Decision making must begin with a simple, mechanical process of association between data and knowledge, conducted without reliance on the practitioner's mind. Thereafter, the processes of care must remain highly organized and explicit. Care would become highly standardized at the front end, and medical decisions at the back end would become highly individualized—precisely the opposite of the status quo, where physicians have broad discretion during the initial patient encounter but are expected to conform to standardized, "evidence-based" guidelines in their ultimate decisions. Enforcing this change makes possible fundamental health care reform at many levels.

III   *The concept of defined inputs.* This part explains the necessity for defined inputs by practitioners. Defining inputs does not mean dictating medical

authored by Dr. Ken Bartholomew, who describes in detail use of knowledge coupling software in conjunction with the POMR in a primary care practice); Weed, LL et al., *Medical Records, Medical Education and Patient Care*, Cleveland: Case Western Reserve University Press (1969); Weed LL. Medical records that guide and teach. *N Engl J Med* 1968 Mar 14;278(11):593-600; Bjorn J, Cross H. *The Problem-Oriented Private Practice of Medicine.* 1970. Chicago: Modern Healthcare Press, pp. 24-28; Burger, Charles S., "The Use of Problem Knowledge Couplers in a Primary Care Practice", *Healthcare Information Management*, vol. 11, no. 4, Winter 1997; C.C. Weed. *The Philosophy, Use and Interpretation of Knowledge Couplers.* PKC Corporation, 1982-2008, available at www.pkc.com; Weed LL, Weed L. Opening the black box of clinical judgment, *British Medical Journal, eBMJ Edition*, Vol 319, issue 7220, 13 November 1999, available at http://bmj.bmjjournals.com/cgi/content/full/319/7220/1279/DC2.

decisions (the direction taken by managed care and evidence-based medicine). Rather, it means enforcing comprehensive standards of performance at a high level, while preserving freedom to exceed those standards. Feedback loops then generate continuous, evolutionary improvements (enforcement against variations for the worse and adoption of variations for the better). This focus on inputs differs fundamentally from current alternatives focused on outcomes or financial incentives or quality indicators. Evidence-based medicine, for example, imposes generalized standards derived from outcomes in large populations, while failing to account for the individual differences that determine outcomes and failing to develop the external tools needed to apply individualized standards.

IV   *Coupling patient data with medical knowledge.* This part focuses on the initial patient workup, where the foundation for care is laid, but the concepts discussed apply more broadly. This part distinguishes between two alternatives—labeled the combinatorial and judgmental approaches—for applying medical knowledge to patient data. Unlike the judgmental approach, the combinatorial approach can be performed by external tools. The basis for choosing between the two approaches is discussed, and "knowledge coupling" tools designed to implement the combinatorial approach are described. See the diagram below, which shows the institutional arrangements within which the tools are built. The combinatorial approach enforces standards of care far more rigorous than accepted medical practice. Physicians object to these standards on various grounds. Answering those objections in detail leads to exploring clinical judgment, the stages of decision making, the nature of medical expertise—in short, the epistemology of medicine. We find that medical practice embodies an unscientific notion of expertise.

V   *Historical and philosophical background:* Pausing from the clinical discussion, this part explores the intellectual behaviors that the combinatorial approach embodies—behaviors that Francis Bacon identified 400 years ago at the birth of modern science. We emphasize a crucial distinction (articulated by Karl Popper) between subjective thought residing in the mind and the objective contents of thought residing in external texts and devices (part V.A). We then tie these issues to F. A. Hayek's analysis of economy of knowledge in market systems, where people constantly avail themselves of knowledge they do not individually possess (part V.B). In health care, people need tools to avail themselves of both knowledge and processing power they do not possess. The tools require simple rules for managing clinical information, just as market systems require accounting standards for managing financial information. This argument views health care as a complex adaptive system, but one that lags centuries behind the evolved systems in the domains of science and commerce.

VI   *The medical record*: Returning to the clinical discussion, this part examines the medical record as a tool for managing detailed patient data over time, after the foundation is laid in the initial workup. The medical record is critical for complex cases involving chronic disease and multiple problems, which is where the largest amount of health care resources are consumed. Medical record standards should be structured to provide simple rules to manage complexity. This means the record should reflect the basic, common-sense steps of orderly problem solving: gathering information, defining problems, formulating plans to address each problem in light of the others, and following through on each plan in light of ongoing feedback. This problem-oriented structure makes possible a unitary medical record for each patient, a record that enables coordinated care by all practitioners, informed involvement by the patient, scientific rigor by clinical researchers, effective scrutiny by third party payers and regulators, and feedback for the total system of care described in the diagram below.

VII   *The nature of medical knowledge as applied to patient care*: This part distinguishes between population-based knowledge about resemblances and patient-specific knowledge about variation among individuals. The latter form of knowledge becomes comprehensible and manageable with new tools and standards for managing information. Moreover, taking into account the medical uniqueness of individuals overcomes the ethical and epistemological limitations of evidence-based medicine. Further, development of medical terminology, taxonomy and coding should be driven not by unstructured clinical judgments of physicians but rather by knowledge coupling tools derived from and linked to a network of medical knowledge that in turn is distilled from the medical literature and continuously improved by analysis of medical records, as diagrammed below.

VIII *Medical education and credentialing*: This part begins by describing how medical schools still fail to integrate clinical and basic science a century after the Flexner Report. Medical education and credentialing must change from a knowledge-based to a skills-based approach. The traditional knowledge-based approach fails to exploit the power of information technology, it completely undermines definition and control of provider inputs to care, and it is educationally harmful. A skills-based approach would use John Dewey's concept of knowledge as a "network of interconnections," embodied in information tools, used by students to access and apply medical knowledge rather than learn it. Learning a core of behavior rather than a core of knowledge, students would be educated from actual experience in patient care. In addition to its educational benefits, this approach would make it possible to rationalize the division of labor in medical practice, further transforming the quality and economics of health care.

IX *Education and the patient/consumer's central role:* This part first analyzes concepts of consumer-driven care, and patient-centered care in the "medical home," arguing that these concepts depend on new tools and standards of care for managing clinical information. Those tools and standards are essential to creating a culture where patients/consumers take responsibility for managing their chronic disease and improving their health behaviors. We argue that patient responsibility requires patient autonomy, which goes beyond the concept of patient-centered care. That discussion leads to the issue of medical education for patients/consumers. Their central role demands that health care should be a subject of formal education from childhood. But formal education, for both practitioners and consumers, must be reformed to break down the usual separation between learning and doing, knowledge and behavior, as John Dewey argued. Health care is the ideal subject matter for applying this reform. From this point of view, we may some day look back on today's school and university education in much the way we look back on alchemy and astrology in the time of Francis Bacon.

Appendix A: Here we analyze two clinical trials of the tools discussed in part IV, concluding that clinical trials have limited value in this context. This Appendix expands on part IV.D, which discusses the problem of evaluating reforms of medical practice.

Appendix B: Here we include a copy of "Scientific principles that tell us why people must manage their own health care," the introduction to a book written for patients in 1975.

The following diagram shows the relationships among the basic components of individualized health care delivery and knowledge development systems.

Individualized Healthcare Delivery and Knowledge Development Systems

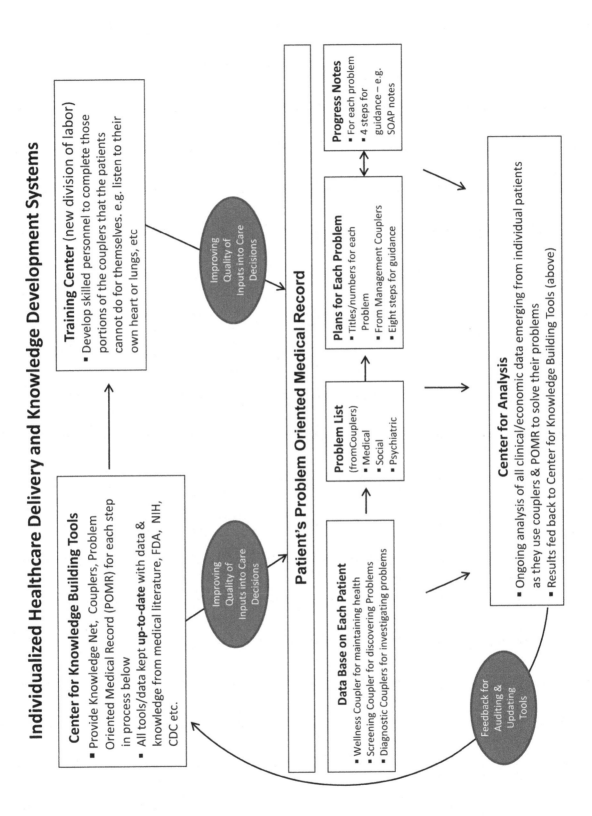

Center for Knowledge Building Tools
- Provide Knowledge Net, Couplers, Problem Oriented Medical Record (POMR) for each step in process below
- All tools/data kept **up-to-date** with data & knowledge from medical literature, FDA, NIH, CDC etc.

Training Center (new division of labor)
- Develop skilled personnel to complete those portions of the couplers that the patients cannot do for themselves. e.g. listen to their own heart or lungs, etc

Improving Quality of Inputs into Care Decisions

Improving Quality of Inputs into Care Decisions

Patient's Problem Oriented Medical Record

Data Base on Each Patient
- Wellness Coupler for maintaining health
- Screening Coupler for discovering Problems
- Diagnostic Couplers for investigating problems

Problem List
(fromCouplers)
- Medical
- Social
- Psychiatric

Plans for Each Problem
- Titles/numbers for each Problem
- From Management Couplers
- Eight steps for guidance

Progress Notes
- For each problem
- 4 steps for guidance – e.g. SOAP notes

Center for Analysis
- Ongoing analysis of all clinical/economic data emerging from individual patients as they use couplers & POMR to solve their problems
- Results fed back to Center for Knowledge Building Tools (above)

Feedback for Auditing & Updating Tools

II.
Disorder and Denial in Medical Practice

A. Failure in medical decision making—a case study

1. Missing an obvious diagnosis

A 1996 *New England Journal of Medicine* case report[3] vividly illustrates medicine's state of denial. The case involved a 15-year-old girl who was admitted to a teaching hospital with a problem of severe fatigue. During months of care this girl almost died, as her undiagnosed condition worsened. Eventually, test results suggested the correct diagnosis—Addison's disease, a deficiency of adrenal-cortical hormones that is fatal if left untreated. This diagnosis was confirmed, and the girl was saved.

Yet, the correct diagnosis in retrospect was "obvious" much earlier, as the article candidly acknowledged. Indeed, several "classic manifestations" of Addison's disease were evident at the initial encounter, and more indications appeared soon after. Nevertheless, multiple physicians missed the diagnosis. In their confusion, they undertook "vastly excessive" testing, which itself was debilitating for their patient.

Their confusion was not surprising. The various manifestations of Addison's disease in this patient are also manifestations of numerous other conditions. Investigating these manifestations would entail considering hundreds of diagnostic possibilities and, for each one, collecting various items of relevant data. Indeed, with respect to this girl's chief complaint of fatigue, review of the medical literature has shown that diagnosis involves taking into account more than 160 diagnostic possibilities—for fatigue and mood disorders (anxiety, depression) often associated with it—and collecting more than 500 items of patient data to determine which of those possibilities are worth considering for

---

3   Keljo D, Squires R. Clinical Problem Solving: Just in Time. *N Engl J Med* 1996: 334:46-48. The discussion here draws on Part I.B of Opening the black box of clinical judgment, note 2 above.

an individual patient.[4] That information goes far beyond what any individual physician can process. In this case, however, the girl's physicians (and the specialists they consulted) acted in denial of this reality. They expected somehow to figure out the correct diagnosis merely from their personal knowledge and judgment. At the most crucial time, the very outset of care, they acted in denial of the need to take into account the full range of diagnostic possibilities and the vast body of knowledge and data made relevant by those possibilities.

Physicians deny that need because they are educated to take into account the limited information their own intellects can comprehend. The alternative is enforcing higher standards of care for managing clinical information, including use of specialized software tools. In this case, for example, use of the necessary standards and tools would have identified Addison's disease as a good match for the girl's signs and symptoms at the initial encounter.[5]

Yet, physicians are not educated to handle complex cases in this manner. Nor are they equipped with the necessary standards, tools, and feedback mechanisms. Instead, they are educated to practice the "art of medicine," using "clinical judgment"—a black box that no one outside the profession can open, a mysterious amalgam of knowledge, analysis and intuition.

This traditional model of practice, of course, is under assault by "evidence-based medicine." But, as we shall see, evidence-based medicine is but a rearrangement of the same broken system. To further describe that system, the next section examines the Addison's disease case in detail.

2. *How it happened*

The report of the Addison's disease case appears in the *New England Journal of Medicine's* "Clinical Problem Solving" series. In these articles, authors present

---

4 This review of the literature has been conducted by PKC Corporation (see the following footnote). The literature review is presented not in journal articles but rather in a new medium—the decision support software referenced in note 2 above. This medium translates knowledge into practice by coupling distilled knowledge with patient data.

5 Versions of the tools referred to have been developed by PKC Corporation. (LLW founded PKC in 1982 and left the company in 2006, due to circumstances not relevant here.) These decision support tools are intended to be used in conjunction with electronic medical record tools (which PKC has also developed), based on the POMR standard (see note 2 above). The PKC versions of these tools are discussed in parts IV.F and VI.D below solely to illustrate the generic concepts and standards that are the subject of this book, not to advocate PKC's particular versions. Any versions of these tools require that the public have confidence in the quality of the information contained in them and confidence in the total system of care of which the tools are a part. The key components of the total system are shown in diagram at the end of Introduction. There needs to be a public discussion of how to build the total system so that the public can use it and trust it just as they use and trust the transportation system.

patient data "in stages" to an expert clinician (referred to as the discussant), who analyzes the data   presented; author commentary follows. Note that patient data are collected and considered piecemeal, "in stages," based on the physician's clinical judgment. This is the traditional approach. A different approach would be first to collect detailed data, defined in advance for the presenting problem, and then consider all of the data *in combination*. The difference between these two approaches is fundamental. Part IV compares these two approaches at length. As background for that comparison, here we review the *New England Journal* article, describing the care the girl received, the authors' analysis of that care, and alternative analyses.

a. Summary of the case

The article begins with data elicited in the first encounter between the 15 year old patient and the doctor who then saw her (no mention is made of reviewing data from prior medical records). The girl had been unable to attend school for three months due to excessive fatigue. For seven months she had experienced weight loss, amenorrhea and shortness of breath on exercise with no wheezing or cough. The physical examination revealed mild hypotension and multiple, deeply pigmented nevi (moles), none with abnormal characteristics. The other findings from the initial history, physical examination and laboratory data were generally normal. The article does not explain the basis for selecting these initial findings. Nor does the article evaluate whether the findings were intelligently selected for diagnosis of the patient's fatigue problem.

The article then describes the discussant's reactions to the initial data. The discussant first observes (correctly) that some of the findings are not seen with chronic fatigue syndrome and suggest an important organic illness. But the discussant does not work through the findings in an organized way. For example, the discussant makes no mention of the girl's nevi, much less inquire whether they first appeared in conjunction with the fatigue problem. Instead, the discussant simply suggests, in a random, incomplete manner, a variety of diagnostic possibilities, most of which are inconsistent in some way with the initial data. For example, the suggestions include hyperthyroidism, but not hypothyroidism, both of which are endocrine disorders for which fatigue is often a symptom. Other endocrine disorders, such as Addison's disease, are unmentioned.

The article then describes how during the next month the girl was admitted to the hospital three times with additional symptoms, including epigastric pain, nausea, bilious emesis, diffuse abdominal pain, diarrhea, dehydration, and further weight loss. Otherwise, her physical examination was unchanged. These findings were consistent with the normal progression of Addison's disease, but that pattern was not recognized. Further gastroenterological examination and testing were undertaken; the article does not indicate the specific rationales for the various tests. Most findings were normal, although some blood test results were borderline. The discussant focused on a finding of *helicobacter pylori* bacteria, recommending treatment but recognizing that this finding would not cause fatigue or amenorrhea.

The girl's undiagnosed condition worsened further as multiple specialists were consulted. They investigated her condition aggressively, generating more and more data to ponder. The girl almost died as she endured "dozens of blood tests, immunologic studies, endoscopies, other radiographic tests and biopsies." During this process, tachycardia (a rapid heart beat) appeared. Several medications were tried. Nasogastric feedings were started and then abandoned after persistent vomiting developed. Intravenous feedings were administered.

A urinalysis showed evidence of ingesting emetine, the active ingredient in ipecac, which bulimics sometimes use to induce vomiting. As often happens when an obvious diagnosis of organic disease is not uncovered, the physicians and the discussant hypothesized psychiatric explanations—bulimia or poisoning by a family member. Despite adamant denials of any ipecac use by the girl and her family, the physicians considered involving child protective services, and they ordered a psychiatric evaluation. An endocrinologist consulted during this period thought that the girl's amenorrhea was consistent with an eating disorder. But this line of investigation was dropped when subsequent tests for emetine were negative (the original test result appeared to be an error), and the psychiatric evaluation did not support the diagnosis of an eating disorder. The article does not indicate whether the girl had any psychiatric symptoms (which often appear during the course of Addison's disease).

Finally, further blood tests revealed abnormal serum electrolyte levels (e.g., hyponatremia, below-normal serum sodium, which initially had been borderline). This development suggested adrenal insufficiency. Further testing confirmed Addison's disease. Hormone replacement therapy was begun, and the girl's condition rapidly improved. "Fortunately," the article observed, "the patient survived not only her illness but the myriad tests and treatments administered before the telltale electrolyte levels revealed the correct diagnosis. Fortunately as well, this happened 'just in time.'"

The article does not explain why electrolyte levels and not earlier findings suggested the correct diagnosis. The discussant concluded that "the only way I could have made the diagnosis earlier is if Addison's disease had been on my differential diagnosis list for anorexia nervosa, but it was not." The reason for this focus on anorexia nervosa is not explained.

Nor does the article explain the rationales for all of the tests and treatments in relation to the various medical problems the girl experienced and the many diagnostic hypotheses considered. One would hope that this information (rationales for actions taken in relation to hypotheses considered) would be explicit in the medical records. In all likelihood, however, the records were ambiguous and incomplete. Unlike experimental scientists recording their data, and unlike businessmen maintaining financial records, physicians typically do not organize medical records in a way that facilitates analysis, communication, and oversight. Medical records for patients do not logically break out the various elements and parameters needed to monitor and manage patient problems. Given this disarray, it is no surprise that "the current diagnostic process in health care is complex, chaotic and vulnerable to failures and breakdowns"—fertile ground for malpractice suits.[6]

As is customary, the article does not describe the economic and psychological realities of a case like this one. The costs incurred, whether third party payers deemed those costs "medically necessary," and the economic burdens of care borne by patients, other payers and their practitioners, are not indicated. Nor does the article describe the emotional impact of the ordeal on the girl and her family.

Similarly, the article does not describe the psychological state of the girl's physicians or the conditions under which their thinking occurred. These factors are highly significant from the perspective of medical decision making. Physicians apply advanced scientific knowledge, but they must do so without the favorable conditions that experimental scientists create for themselves. Multitasking is forced on physicians, often in chaotic environments and under severe time and resource constraints. Physicians may not choose the problems to investigate, the variables to consider and the conditions in which to perform. In this case, for example, we can assume that all of the physicians were coping with

---

6 Gandhi T., et al. Missed and Delayed Diagnoses in the Ambulatory Setting: A Study of Closed Malpractice Claims, *Ann Intern Med* 2006; 145:488-496 (Oct. 3, 2006). See also Gandhi T, Lee T. Patient Safety beyond the Hospital. *New Eng. J. Med.* 363:1001-1003 (Sept. 8, 2010) ("Practices are now observing that missed or delayed diagnoses are the most common problem leading to malpractice claims in the outpatient setting"), at http://www.nejm.org/doi/full/10.1056/NEJMp1003294. The CRICO Harvard Risk Management Foundation states: "Missed, delayed, or incorrect diagnoses account for approximately one-quarter of all malpractice cases naming CRICO-insured providers," based on 1,134 claims asserted from 2005-2009. http://www.rmf.harvard.edu/high-risk-areas/diagnosis/index.aspx.

many patients, some of greater complexity than this girl, and some presenting issues outside each physician's training, experience and specialty interest.

Patients trust that all their medical needs will be taken into account and skillfully managed, but no physician has the range of knowledge and skills needed to fulfill that trust. Yet, physicians find it hard to acknowledge this reality, even to themselves. Moreover, physicians are often held responsible for harmful outcomes beyond their control, while functioning in conditions of disorder they feel powerless to change. The result is that physicians bear terrible psychological burdens. In addition to the threat of unfair malpractice litigation, they live with the constant risk of harming their own patients, and are haunted by memories of their own errors. Over time, the emotional burdens they carry may increasingly impair their functioning. These factors likely contribute to unusually high rates of depression, substance abuse and suicide among physicians.[7]

b. The article's analysis

Summarizing the girl's condition during her care, the article candidly describes the perplexity of her physicians, the consultants and the discussant:

> At one time or another, the unfortunate child described here suffered from weakness, breathlessness, abdominal pain, nausea, vomiting, diarrhea, weight loss, and severe malnutrition. Examination never disclosed any findings other than tachycardia, mild hypotension and dehydration. Neither the patient's physician and several consultants nor the discussant considered the correct diagnosis—Addison's disease—on the basis of these clinical findings. Yet the diagnosis became obvious as soon as hyponatremia, hyperkalemia and hypobicarbonatemia developed months after her initial presentation. . . .

That summary implies that the diagnostic delay was not readily avoidable. "A rare diagnosis that is obvious in retrospect," the authors observe, "is often not so obvious prospectively." In support of their view, the authors cite two difficulties presented by this case:

- The initial "classic manifestations" of Addison's disease in this patient were not specific to that condition. Findings such as fatigue, hypotension, dehydration, and dermatologic abnormalities suggest innumerable diagnostic possibilities.

---

7   See Leape L, Fromson J. Problem Doctors: Is There a System Solution? *Ann Intern Med* 2006. 144: 107-115; Schernhammer E. Taking Their Own Lives: The High Rate of Physician Suicide, *New Eng J Med* 2005, 354;24:2473-2476.

- The presentation of Addison's disease in this patient seemed atypical. Reportedly, the disease is especially rare in teenage girls, amenorrhea does not usually appear, the initially normal blood electrolytes levels are uncharacteristic of Addison's disease, and the girl's nevi differed from the "more classic dermatologic changes" expected with the disease. (None of the physicians apparently considered these points during the girl's care, but the authors raise these points in trying to explain why the possibility of Addison's disease did not occur to anyone.)

The article does not discuss whether these difficulties are frequently encountered in patient care. But the article does discuss what happens when patients do not conform to physician beliefs about what is specific or typical:

Disaster lurks when a patient has a life-threatening disease that not only is rare but also presents with either atypical or non-specific symptoms or signs. In patients with diseases that fit this description, vastly excessive testing and numerous attempts to treat putative diagnoses are the rule. We can be certain that in such instances some patients die because the correct diagnosis is never entertained and that even after an autopsy the mystery persists.[8]

An unexamined premise here is the validity of physician beliefs about specific or typical findings. The authors do not consider the possibility that non-specific findings might be highly specific *in combination*. Nor do the authors consider the possibility that "atypical" variation from typical findings is routine, not unusual. Nor do they consider whether medical "knowledge" of what is typical overlooks the many cases never examined by researchers and the many cases where relevant findings were never checked or never intelligibly recorded, not to mention those cases where the correct diagnosis was never even entertained. From their limited perspective, the authors go on to observe:

---

8   For other reports of undiagnosed Addison's disease, see Bird S., "Failure to diagnose: Addison's disease." *Australian Family Physician*, 58:859-861 (October 2007) (death of a 16 year old girl), available at http://www.racgp.org.au/afp/200710/19347. See also http://www.bmj.com/cgi/eletters/319/7220/1279 (quoting a personal communication from the father of a 10 year boy who died of Addison's disease, where that condition was suspected but not tested for); Boodman, S. A piece of presidential history solved the puzzle. Washington Post, Dec. 15, 1999 (various physicians missed Addison's disease for eight months, until one of them notice the patient's hyperpigmentation and had "a hunch triggered by photographs she'd seen of a ruddy-looking President John F. Kennedy, who had Addison's disease"), available at http://www.washingtonpost.com/wp-dyn/content/article/2009/12/14/AR2009121402863.html.

... When a patient's findings are nonspecific—as they were in this instance—the number of diagnostic possibilities is often enormous, and *the clinician usually begins his diagnostic investigation by considering (and excluding) the most common diagnoses.* As these most common diagnoses become less likely, many less common diagnoses are considered. Unfortunately, in this case Addison's disease did not make the list until it was nearly too late to save the child's life. [Emphasis added.]

Here, an unexamined premise is that the usual approach (considering first "the most common diagnoses") is sound. Accepting that premise, the authors seem to believe that the diagnostic struggle in this unusual case was to be expected. "Only the toughest critic could fault any of the clinicians for not making the correct diagnosis earlier ...." The authors' further conclusions are narrow and disappointing:

we would be irresponsible if we failed to learn a lesson from this patient. Addison's disease is rare in [patients like this one]. ... Nonetheless, as this case illustrates, Addison's disease, though rare, does occur and can be present for long periods without its classic manifestations.[9] Perhaps the only way to have made this diagnosis earlier would have been to appreciate that none of the diagnoses entertained by any of the physicians involved in the patient's care explained all of the clinical findings. *At that point*, a resourceful physician might have explored *exhaustive lists* of conditions that—no matter how *rare and atypical*—might be responsible. [Emphasis added.]

These conclusions raise several basic questions that the article does not consider. What does "rare and atypical" mean when considering an individual instead of a population? Should software tools instead of resourceful physicians be used to generate "exhaustive lists" of diagnostic possibilities? Should that thoroughness be a first step instead of a last resort?

c. A different analysis

Notwithstanding its apparent conclusion that an early diagnosis was difficult, the article provides many clues suggesting just the opposite. "In retrospect, the diagnosis seems obvious. *Fatigue, weakness, dehydration and hypotension are classic manifestations of Addison's disease*" (emphasis added). At least three of these telltale findings were made at the initial encounter (the dehydration

---

9   Here the article contradicts its prior acknowledgement of "classic manifestations" early in the case.

finding was made ten days later, but one wonders if it was present initially and not checked). Also observed at the outset was another classic manifestation— unusual skin pigmentation. "Multiple practitioners commented on the patient's large number of deeply pigmented nevi, and there is a report of such changes in Addison's disease."[10] Whether or not atypical, these nevi could have been recognized as a possible variation on the reportedly "more classic dermatologic changes" expected to appear with Addison's disease. In addition, this patient manifested further signs of the disease within the first month of care, including the dehydration, nausea, abdominal pain and malnutrition, all of which are quite typical of the disease. Despite this compelling body of evidence, the possibility of Addison's disease did not even occur to the various physicians involved for months, "until it was nearly too late to save the child's life."

As noted, the authors attribute this delay to the nonspecific nature of the initial findings and the seemingly atypical presentation of the disease in this girl. Yet, to reiterate, so-called non-specific findings, when considered *in combination*, may be highly specific. That is why *common* findings like fatigue, hypotension and dehydration are "classic manifestations" of a *rare* condition like Addison's disease. Moreover, the presentation of the disease in this girl was more typical than the authors suggest. The initially borderline serum sodium level should have been seen as below normal in the context of dehydration. The "large number of deeply pigmented nevi" should have been seen as a reported variant of the hyperpigmentation that is known to be an early manifestation of Addison's disease. More broadly, variations from the expected should be seen as the rule, not the exception. That is, unique individual variations should be seen collectively as no less common than the so-called classic case, and no less important to take into account at the outset of care.

Individual variation is perceived as normal when occurring in faces and physiques. In physiology and pathology, variation is equally normal and pervasive. Yet, it is often perceived as abnormal, or is not perceived at all. The reason is that medical knowledge about physiology and pathology is usually expressed as rough generalizations about large populations. Knowledge expressed in that form is more easily recalled and processed by the unaided mind than detailed data about unique individual variations. As a result, these more detailed data are less likely to be incorporated in the body of medical knowledge (that is, less likely to be published or otherwise made generally available). Even when thus incorporated in medical knowledge, detailed information about unique

---

10   Authors' reply to letters to the editor, N Eng J Med. 1996;334:1404-1405, citing Ibsen HH, Clemmenson O. Eruptive Nevi in Addison's disease. Arch Dermatol 1990; 126:1239-40 (describing a patient in Denmark).

individual cases is less likely to be taken into account by practitioners, because their unaided minds cannot quickly comb through the medical literature. In the Addison's disease case, for example, none of the multiple practitioners who commented on their patient's deeply pigmented nevi were aware of an article on a Addison's disease patient in Denmark with nevi of similar appearance (see note 10 above). (It is unknown how frequently Addison's disease manifests itself with this form of hyperpigmentation, in part because medical records do not reliably record such data, in part because records are not maintained in a structured electronic form accessible to researchers, and in part because Addison's disease sometimes occurs without ever being diagnosed.)

In short, the unaided mind naturally turns to population-based medical knowledge. Yet that knowledge falls far short of what is needed for the care of unique individuals. The more individualized knowledge that patients need is either unknown or not accessible. This shortfall is most critical at the outset of care. As the case study observes, clinicians usually begin diagnostic investigation by considering first population-based knowledge of what diagnose are "most common." (Thus the aphorism among physicians—"when you hear hoof beats, think horses, not zebras.") Yet, this approach is fraught with risk, because it may divert attention from the diagnostic possibilities most applicable to the individual patient. In the case study, for example, Addison's disease, a rare condition, "did not make the list [of diagnoses to consider] until it was nearly too late to save the child's life." Whether a disease is common or rare depends on the context. (Thus the aphorism among physicians might become, in central Africa, "when you hear hoof beats, think zebras, not horses."). In the general population, Addison's disease is indeed rare. But in the tiny subpopulation of patients with a combination of findings like fatigue, hypotension, weight loss, abnormal pigmentation, dehydration, nausea, and abdominal pain, Addison's disease is *common* (perhaps almost universal). People with this pattern of findings are not identified as a subpopulation in the medical literature and thus do not fit into the usual "evidence-based" mode of analysis.

As applied to individuals, knowledge about large populations is useless, indeed misleading, until other, more individually applicable knowledge is first taken into account. Yet, this other, individualized knowledge is not made readily accessible. Even more disturbing is the health care establishment's response to this dilemma. Physicians are increasingly expected to apply knowledge derived from large population studies and clinical trials. Referred to as "evidence-based medicine," a better label for this approach would be "evidence-missed medicine," because it systematically excludes the individualized knowledge and data essential to patient care. Yet, "so-called evidence-based medicine is rapidly becoming the canon in many hospitals," Dr. Jerome Groopman observes. "Treatments outside the statistically proven are considered taboo until a sufficient body of data can be collected from clinical trials."[11]

Evidence-based medicine is rightly intended to prevent physicians from following arbitrary local practices and unsupported personal judgments. But that goal can only be achieved by meticulous accounting for individualized information. Absence of that basic standard of care explains the delayed diagnosis in the Addison's disease case and much of the health care system's dysfunction.

d. Further analyses from readers

The points in the above analysis were not addressed in any of the numerous letters to the editor published by the *New England Journal* in response to the case study. The letters expressed opposing views on whether the physicians were at fault for not diagnosing the girl's condition earlier. A variety of clinical analyses were suggested, with no consensus on how the case should have been handled.

A primary source of confusion in cases like this one is that physicians tend to think within specialty boundaries. Yet, patient problems usually cross those boundaries. The various specialties generate a corresponding variety of clinical analyses. This variety is most apparent when patients have multiple co-morbid conditions, but it also occurs with a single condition. To illustrate, Addison's disease is an endocrine disorder that manifests itself with metabolic, gastrointestinal, cardiovascular, dermatologic and psychiatric symptoms and signs, which appear in variable ways over time in different patients. In this case, one of the consultants was an endocrinologist, but he missed the diagnosis in his own specialty. The specialty of the authors and apparently of the discussant (gastroenterology) seemed to heavily influence their thinking. One of the correspondents criticized the authors in this regard, but that correspondent proposed an exceedingly indirect cardiovascular analysis, ignoring more obvious indications of Addison's disease. As the authors observed in response, "clinicians work from short lists, and these lists vary from specialty to specialty."[12]

The letters to the editor, like the article itself, suggest that medical decision making is an intellectual Tower of Babel. This confusion is especially disturbing when one considers that this case was relatively simple, and occurred under favorable conditions. The patient had a single, identifiable disease with relatively few abnormalities to investigate, and she received care at a teaching hospital where expert specialists were readily available. Moreover, critical findings were available at an early stage, established knowledge was sufficient for the patient

---

11 Groopman J. *How Doctors Think* (New York: Houghton Mifflin, 2007), pp. 5-6.
12 Authors' reply to letters to the editor, N Eng J Med. 1996;334:1404-1405.

to be diagnosed quickly, and a clear, efficacious treatment for the diagnosis was known. If physicians are unable to apply established knowledge effectively in a simple case like this one, then what hope is there for complex patients, where multiple problems are present, where those problems interact and evolve in highly individualized ways, where intricate data collection and analysis over time is required, where the data may not fit with established knowledge, where medical interventions may further complicate analysis, where uncertain diagnostic possibilities or treatment options must be assessed, or where risky and invasive procedures may be unavoidable? In many such cases, especially cases of chronic illness, the difficulties are further heightened by the fact that patient's active and informed involvement is essential, and everything that happens must be communicated among multiple practitioners and organizations for months or years.

The heart of the problem is that physicians are trained to rely on their personal judgment about what data to collect and what the data mean. The obvious alternative to personal judgment is software guidance tools. But software tools accomplish little if they are designed merely to mimic physician judgment. Because of the mind's limited information processing capacity, judgment relies on cognitive shortcuts. Software tools should be designed to avoid those shortcuts, and take full advantage of the computer's huge capacity for raw information processing.

Illustrating what software should *not* do, one of the letters to the editor about the Addison's disease case described the results that a diagnostic decision support software product would have generated, based on data entered in the order presented by the article. "After the data obtained during the initial history and physical examination were entered, the list of diagnoses proposed by the system *focused, as did the physicians, on (relatively) common disorders*, such as anorexia nervosa and Graves' disease" (emphasis added). The initial output thus completely missed the correct diagnosis, even though classic manifestations of Addison's disease were among the initial data. The next round of data entry enabled the software to identify Addison's disease, but not to highlight it among many other diagnostic possibilities. After the third round of data entry, Addison's disease was ranked second on the list of diagnostic possibilities.[13] Although an improvement over the physicians, the software's performance was unimpressive.

13 "When the epigastric pain and nausea and all the normal initial basic laboratory test results were entered, chronic pancreatitis and several lymphomas moved to the top of the list, with chronic adrenal insufficiency now appearing as number 17. When I added the vomiting, the dehydration, and the second round of laboratory tests, Addison's disease moved up to number 2—well before this disease was considered by the physicians caring for the patient or by the discussant." Hoffer E. N Eng J Med. 1996;334:1404 [letters]

Clearly, something different is required from software tools than attempting to reproduce clinical judgment.

A more impressive diagnostic performance is described in another letter to the editor. This correspondent became "dissatisfied with the reasoning of the discussant in the first paragraph" and stopped reading the article after 3½ paragraphs. He started again by constructing his own differential diagnosis. Relying solely on the symptoms and signs from the initial history and physical examination (before lab results), this correspondent "came to just one possibility—Addison's disease." He criticized the physicians and the discussant for (1) overlooking a clue to the diagnosis in the patient's circulatory condition, (2) using data selectively to support hypotheses while neglecting contradictory or absent data inconsistent with the hypotheses, and (3) failing "to start again at the very beginning of the diagnostic process" after their initial perplexity, when it became apparent that they needed to follow "the basic systematics of data collection and evaluation."[14]

This conclusion raises some fundamental questions. What exactly is meant by "the basic systematics of data collection and evaluation"? Do these practices mean limited data collection targeted at limited number of diagnostic hypotheses, determined by the practitioner's judgment? Or do these practices mean detailed data collection covering a broad range of diagnostic possibilities for the patient's problem, without introducing the practitioner's judgment? In either case, how can these practices be defined, disseminated and enforced? To what extent can these practices be captured in software guidance tools for use by all practitioners and patients themselves, with less dependence on the scarce, expensive and unreliable services of highly educated physicians? We address those and related questions in relation to the initial patient encounter (part IV) and the subsequent processes of care (part VI). First, however, in part II.B we further examine implications of the case study for reform of medical practice, and in part III we examine a basic principle essential to overcoming the health care system's pervasive disorder.

In considering what follows, the reader should understand that front-line physicians are not to blame for the disorder in which they find themselves.[15] On the contrary, physicians are waging a daily struggle to overcome that disorder. But all too often their efforts are unequal to the task, even in cases where favorable

---

14   De Loos W. N Eng J Med. 1996;334:1403 [letters]

15   In particular, the physicians involved in the Addison's disease case are not to be blamed for the broken system of care the case study describes. To their credit, the two physicians who authored the article did not present the favorable outcome as a success story. Instead, they recognized that a serious problem existed, and they candidly described the problem for others to learn from.

outcomes ultimately occur. Some favorable outcomes, as in the case study, are achieved at unacceptable risk, suffering and cost. Some favorable outcomes occur independently of medical intervention or in spite of it, because of the body's remarkable homeostatic mechanisms for self-repair. Where physician efforts do result in optimal care, those achievements are more personal than systemic. Missing is a system of order and transparency in which to invest remarkable scientific advances and the enormous personal efforts of practitioners. Were those scientific and personal resources invested more effectively, then health care might become as productive as other information-intensive, technologically-advanced endeavors. Were there a system of order and transparency, health care might become an arena of continuous improvement, rather than a quagmire of intractable dilemmas—a source of hope for our economic future, rather than its greatest threat.

B. Implications for reform of medical practice

1. Medicine's division of intellectual labor

Medical decision making requires sorting through a vast body of available information to identify the limited information actually needed for each patient. That individually-relevant information must be applied reliably and efficiently, without unnecessary trial and error. This requires highly organized analysis. Educated guesswork is not good enough.

Organized analysis can begin with a simple process of association. In the diagnostic context, this means linking a symptom with associated diagnoses, linking each one of those diagnostic possibilities with readily observable, inexpensive findings associated with each diagnosis, checking all of those findings in the patient, and comparing actual, positive findings on the patient with the array of diagnostic possibilities and associated findings. The output of this process reveals how well each of the diagnostic possibilities matches the patient. (Such a process of association should similarly form the basis for selecting among different treatment possibilities, as we shall see.)

This process of association is simple in two senses. First, the data items are quick, inexpensive, non-invasive findings from the patient history, physical examination and basic laboratory tests. Second, no clinical judgment is required to establish the simple associations between the findings and the diagnoses. The associations (distilled from the medical literature) are mere linkages that computer software can instantly arrange and rearrange as needed.

Physicians are not trained to begin diagnosis using external tools for this simple associative process. Instead, they employ clinical judgment from the very outset of care. Somehow, at each encounter with a new patient, physicians must rapidly select the right data, and then analyze that data correctly in light of vast medical knowledge. They believe that their judgment organizes data collection and analysis in a scientifically sophisticated manner (referred to as "differential diagnosis" in the diagnostic context). This is believed superior to mere information processing, because it applies scientific knowledge and, when successful, minimizes unnecessary data collection. An example is the correspondent (discussed in the preceding section) who analyzed very limited initial data in the case study and "came to just one possibility—Addison's disease." Moreover, clinical judgment involves observation and intuition based on personal interaction with the patient, informed by long experience with innumerable other patients. Physicians thus believe that clinical judgment involves much more than educated guesswork.

Yet, it is a fantasy to think that clinical judgment enables physicians to analyze patient problems reliably and efficiently. After all, the various physicians in the case study failed to do so. So did the discussant, and so did all but one of the correspondents submitting letters to the editor. Moreover, their perplexity cannot be dismissed as mere incompetence, unrepresentative of medical practice. On the contrary, the article describing their perplexity was accepted by one of the leading medical journals in the world. And that article offered no clear solution to the diagnostic difficulties it described. Nor did the one correspondent who arrived at the correct diagnosis from the initial data. His admonition to follow the "basic systematics of data collection and evaluation" is not a defined, reproducible and enforceable solution. And we cannot be confident that this physician would be equally successful in other cases. He analyzed a medical journal article, not an actual patient in real time. Moreover, his personal knowledge happened to match well with the case. That would not always occur, because there is no single core of knowledge enabling physicians to analyze all patient problems (which is one reason why physicians specialize). Even if such a core of knowledge could be established, not all physicians would learn it completely or keep it current. Moreover, physicians operating under the difficult conditions of patient care are not always able to apply correctly whatever knowledge they happen to possess. Many talented physicians thus "find that the skills that allowed them to excel in the classroom, and even as house officers, are of little use in their medical careers."[16]

Any system of care that depends on the personal knowledge and analytic capacities of physicians cannot be trusted. And even if basic information processing by physicians could somehow be improved to the point where it is trustworthy, the supply of physicians would remain scarce and expensive. It

---

16   Shaughnessy A, Slawson D. Are we providing doctors with the training and tools for lifelong learning? *BMJ* 1999; 319; 1280.

is a utopian fantasy to think that health care will ever be universally reliable, affordable, and accessible if highly educated, highly compensated physicians are always essential to its delivery.

The traditional concept of the learned physician is not workable. The concept is that applying advanced medical science requires practitioners who have passed through an extraordinarily prolonged and expensive ordeal of education, apprenticeship and credentialing. But precisely the opposite is the case. Medical training in its current form is not only unnecessary but incompatible with scientific rigor. Applying complex medical science to unique patients in all their infinite variety under real-world time constraints demands information processing beyond the capacity of anyone, no matter how gifted, well schooled or experienced. And that would be true even in a best-case scenario where all physicians performed at their peak. Many physicians perform at less than their peak, not only those who succumb to depression and substance abuse (see note 7 above) but also those who are coping with impossible burdens.

A new division of labor is required. Medical decision making should begin with a simple process of association, carried out with digital information tools. From that foundation, the informed mind can then apply judgment, intuition and personal values. This division of labor is liberating for both practitioners and patients. Physicians are freed from the prohibitive burden of raw information processing, and thereby freed to master hands-on skills. Non-physician practitioners are freed from physician authority over medical information processing. Patients are freed from dependence on physicians for access to the information they need to make personal choices about their own bodies and minds. Practitioners and patients alike become better equipped to make human judgments that should not be entrusted to external tools.

Nevertheless, for some physicians this new division of labor may appear to be not liberating but dispiriting. Non-physicians practitioners and patients themselves using external information tools will invade intellectual territory that has always been the private preserve of the medical profession. That change threatens not only the profession's authority but its ideal of itself. Dr. Sherwin Nuland has articulated that ideal:

> To understand pathophysiology is to hold the key to diagnosis, without which there can be no cure. The quest of every doctor in approaching serious disease is to make the diagnosis and to design and carry out the specific cure. This quest I call The Riddle, and I capitalize it so there will be no mistaking its dominance over every other consideration. The satisfaction of solving The Riddle is its own reward, and the fuel that

drives the clinical engines of medicine's most highly trained specialists. It is every doctor's measure of his own abilities; it is the most important ingredient in his professional self-image. ... Our most rewarding moments of healing derive not from the works of our hearts but from those of our intellects – it is there that the passion is most intense.[17]

This passion now pursues a misguided ideal of intellectual virtuosity. But once the passion is pursued with the aid of external information tools, it becomes more interesting, more rewarding, more sustainable, more available to *all* practitioners and more connected to patient needs. And that connection to patients is what medical practice is ultimately about.

Other fields of expertise have found that external tools do not destroy what is best in those fields. Beryl Markham discussed this phenomenon in her reminiscences about flying. On the attitude of an older pilot who resisted instrument-controlled flying, she wrote:

After this era of great pilots has gone, as the era of great sea captains has gone – each nudged aside by the march of inventive genius, by steel cogs and copper discs and hand thin wires on white faces that are dumb, but speak—it will be found, I think, that all the science of flying has been captured on the breadth of an instrument board, but not the religion of it.[18]

The religion of medicine is not feats of intellect. The religion of medicine is helping to solve the problems of patients, and the compassion involved in the very act of care. But helping patients in the name of caring or compassion may do more harm than good, if the help is not competent. And competence in the face of complexity requires practitioners to use external tools, tools "that are dumb, but speak."

2. Implications of changing medicine's division of labor

a. The significance of information technology

Rethinking the division of labor reveals why digital information technology has created a turning point in medicine's history. Just as microscopes made it possible to observe disease at the cellular level, so the right information technology now makes it possible to apply vast medical knowledge to detailed patient data with reliability and speed.

17   Nuland, Sherwin B. *How We Die: Reflections of Life's Final Chapter* (NewYork: Alfred A. Knopf, 1994), pp. 248-49.

18   Markham, B., *West With the Night* (San Francisco: Both Point Press, 1983), p. 186.

This potential for digital information processing to advance medical decision making is obvious. Perhaps less obvious is the potential to advance medical knowledge itself. Just as instruments like the microscope and the telescope revealed whole new worlds for observation in science, so instruments for processing information can radically expand the scope of usable knowledge and data for comprehension in medicine. Increasingly, medical knowledge will encompass not just generalizations about large populations (a form of knowledge relatively accessible to the unaided mind) but also enormously detailed understanding about the infinite variety of unique individuals (a form of knowledge the mind needs external aids to comprehend). Coping with this complexity is becoming more and more essential, as genomics and proteomics are creating detailed new data about every individual and correspondingly intricate bodies of knowledge (see part VII).

The culture of medicine has yet to confront these realities. Physician training, credentialing and functioning remain fundamentally unchanged—even though cognitive error in medicine is now recognized as epidemic, even though consensus has developed on the need for electronic medical records and other "health information technology," even though health care institutions increasingly use digital technologies for storing, retrieving and communicating information, even though practitioners and patients use the Internet to gain unprecedented access to medical knowledge, and even though health information networks are being developed to permit interoperability among disparate systems and institutions. Despite these advances, the physician's mind remains heavily burdened with the core function of processing information—applying comprehensive general knowledge to inform selection and analysis of patient-specific data—even as the new technologies accelerate information overload. This is a burden too great for the human mind to bear.

Placing this burden on the mind completely undermines order and transparency in medical decision making. The mind is variable, idiosyncratic, inefficient, unreliable and opaque when attempting to process detailed information on the fly. Unavoidably, the mind introduces disorder. As the case study illustrates, that disorder occurs from the beginning of the initial encounter with a new patient, undermining everything that follows. And that disorder is intractable, because the mind's internal functioning is not subject to scrutiny and control.

The disorder introduced by misplaced reliance on the human mind compromises the various uses of information technology enumerated above. In every field, and especially in medicine, information technology alone is no remedy for disorder in underlying work processes.[19] Effective use of information technology demands rigorous standards of care for managing medical information. Standards are needed in two core areas (the subjects of parts IV and VI below): (1) selection and analysis of patient data based on medical knowledge, and (2) using medical records to organize data generated by patient care over time. As long as disorder in these two areas is tolerated, the enormous potential of health information technology in medicine will remain unfulfilled.

b. The nature of disorder in medical decision making

Disorder is apparent to any patient who brings the same medical problem to different physicians. One would hope that their scientific training would cause different physicians each to follow established standards for initial investigation of a given problem, including careful documentation of positive and negative findings. But this is not what happens. The patient is virtually certain to find that different physicians collect different bodies of information, even though presented with the same problem in the same person. Little uniformity exists in taking a history, doing a physical examination and ordering laboratory tests.[20] Moreover, as the case study illustrates, different physicians may well draw different inferences even when they consider the same data and even when only one conclusion is supportable from medical knowledge. This remarkable variation reflects medicine's lack of standards for initial investigation of specific medical problems, lack of dissemination and enforcement even when standards exist, and lack of any mechanism for assuring that data will be assessed correctly. This lack of standards results in variation in how different providers approach the same patient—which is far more significant than variation in how different providers approach the "same" disease condition in different patients (see parts IV.G.3 and VII below).

---

19 "To gain the most benefits from any significant information systems project, an organization must focus its attention on process redesign. … Healthcare … may represent an extreme case of the importance of this principle." See PricewaterhouseCoopers, "Reactive to Adaptive: Transforming Hospitals with Digital Technology," March 2005, p. 11, available at http://www.isedis.com/documents/Price-Waterhouse%20Digital%20Hospitals.pdf. See also pp. 29-31.

20 As to lab tests, Dr. George Lundberg has estimated that "about 80 percent of the tests carried out in the laboratories I oversaw in academic medical centers did not need to be done." He also describes studies of arbitrary physician ordering behavior, and observes: "doctors' examinations are now almost superseded by batteries of tests. When we look at why physicians order tests, we discover a wide variety of reasons, but few of them have anything to do with science." In one of the studies cited by Dr. Lundberg, the volume of orders of two expensive tests was reduced by two thirds and one third merely by changing the hospital lab request form. ("Just as most diners rarely order something that is not on the menu, so doctors rarely order tests not listed on the test request slip.") Lundberg, G. *Severed Trust: Why American Medicine Hasn't Been Fixed* (New York: Basic Books, 2000), pp. 22, 257-59.

Similar disorder appears when doctors record their activities in medical records, whether paper or electronic. Medicine does not enforce rational standards for recording physicians' data collection, assessment and follow-up. Indeed, medical records are so variable in structure and completeness that it is often impossible to reliably trace connections among the data collected, the patient's problems, the physician's assessments, the actions taken, the patient's behaviors, the patient's progress and ultimate outcomes. Electronic records do not remedy these failings, and may make them worse. The disorganization of medical records both reflects and exacerbates disorganization in how physicians manage patient care over time, especially the care of complex patients with chronic disease and multiple problems. This disorder makes patient care fragmentary, uncoordinated and rife with error and waste. And it prevents medical records from being an intelligible or trustworthy source of data for outcome comparisons and clinical research.

Instead of defining rigorous standards of care in these matters, medicine gives free rein to the autonomous physician's clinical judgment. Yet, the exercise of clinical judgment defies organized quality improvement. Stated differently, internal cognitive functioning is not subject to scrutiny and control unless it is made defined and explicit.

A useful comparison is standards of accounting for financial information. Centuries before digital information technologies existed, accounting standards created a framework for order and transparency in financial information (see part V.B below). Without the framework provided by accounting standards, complex business enterprises would defy comprehension and control. The Enron debacle and other cases like it demonstrate the disorder that occurs when accounting standards are not enforced.

In the financial world, standards of accounting are generally accepted. Failure to enforce those standards in cases like Enron is thus a scandal. In medicine the scandal is larger. Necessary standards are not even recognized in medicine, much less generally accepted or enforced. It is as if businesses prepared financial statements without regard to established concepts of assets, liabilities, revenue, expenses and double-entry bookkeeping. In medicine, analogous departures from rational standards of care contribute to the opaque, uncoordinated, out-of-control non-system of care that practitioners and patients cope with every day.[21]

---

21 Ninety years ago, a pioneer of qualify improvement in medicine, Ernest Amory Codman, observed that hospital trustees require audits of financial accounts but feel no duty to similarly audit the work of medical staff. *A Study in Hospital Efficiency* (privately published, 1918), p. 12. Now, the work of medical providers is subject to intense micromanagement by third party payers. But this intervention is too often not clinically credible, because medicine is practiced without basic accounting standards for clinical information.

No practitioner has the comprehensive expertise needed to evaluate or provide what each patient individually needs. So various experts are consulted, almost at random, in the hope some of their expertise might match patient needs. Many of the services provided by practitioners are highly complex and costly, with the potential for unintended harmful consequences, which in turn set in motion more dangerous and costly activity. Moreover, all this activity is poorly understood and coordinated by multiple practitioners, the patient, and the patient's family.[22] None are equipped with the tools and standards to manage the complexity they face. Financial forces are thus left free to infect decision making by default.

As Dr. Sandeep Jauhaur has written, after describing the care of a hospital patient who was seen by 17 specialists and underwent 12 procedures in one month: "where doctors are paid piecework for their services, if you have a slew of physicians and a willing patient, almost any sort of terrible excess can occur."[23] Equally terrible *deprivation* of care can occur where doctors are paid a fixed amount per patient (capitation).[24] The common element in both situations is the lack of systems that give all parties involved an objective view of patients' medical needs, in the way that accounting systems provide an objective view of a company's financial position.

To reiterate, merely introducing information technology into this disorder accomplishes little. New information tools are essential, but their design and use must be informed by new standards of care. Equally important, the medical content built into those tools must be subjected to rigorous feedback and continuous improvement from controlled experience recorded in structured medical records. In contrast, the medical content built into the minds of

---

22   See Bodenheimer, T. Coordinating Care — A Perilous Journey through the Health Care System. *New Eng. J. Med.* 358:10; 1064-1071 (March 6, 2008).

23   Jauhar S. "Many Doctors, Many Tests, No Rhyme or Reason," *The New York Times*, March 11, 2008. Dr. Jauhar's essay generated remarkable commentary from many readers, both patients and practitioners, who further described the lack of "rhyme or reason" in medical services. See http://community.nytimes.com/article/comments/2008/03/11/health/views/11essa.html?s=1&pg=1.

24   Malcolm Sparrow, an expert on fraud and fraud control, has written, "the introduction of capitated or prospective payment systems [to avoid fraud in fee-for-service systems] carries with it an entirely new set of problems and new fraud types; these are considerably more dangerous to human health than the traditional fee-for-service frauds." *License to Steal: How Fraud Bleeds America's Health Care System* (Westview Press, updated edition, 2000), pp. 53-54. Sparrow sees this danger as one of a number of drawbacks of shifting from fee-for-service to standardized payment systems. "As we learn more about the new problems introduced by the inversion of the financial incentives, it becomes all the more imperative to learn how to run a fee-for-service system well without being knocked down repeatedly by wave after waive of fraud." *Ibid.*, pp. 54-55.

physicians is unstable, unreliable, unknown to others and not subject to organized feedback and improvement.

The elements of disorder discussed so far relate to medical decision making. Disorder is equally pervasive in execution of medical decisions. At that stage of care, medical error and threats to patient safety are epidemic. This issue has deservedly become prominent within the last decade. We will return to the issue of decision execution when we discuss defined inputs in part III and medical education in part VIII.

c. Basic implications for health care reform

Bringing order and transparency to medical practice would cause its formative social institutions—graduate medical education, credentialing systems, reimbursement entitlements and the doctor-patient relationship—to undergo wrenching transformations. Already the doctor-patient relationship is in upheaval, because the Internet gives patients unprecedented access to medical knowledge. But that disruption falls short of a genuine transformation, because it does not remove the source of disorder—dependence on the unaided human mind for information processing. A genuine transformation would begin by breaking this dependence—a logjam at the center of the health care system. It would go on to transform how medical knowledge is coupled with patient data, how the fragmentary processes of care are organized around patient problems, how and by whom medical decisions are made, how the systems and processes for executing decisions are designed, how new medical knowledge is harvested from patient care and how practitioners are trained and credentialed.

These transformations in medical practice are the foundation for other dimensions of health care reform, in particular the goal of universal coverage. Universal coverage will never be economically viable until it delivers value commensurate with the resources invested in it.[25] If medical practice remains in its present state of disorder, universal coverage will be no more affordable than homeownership financed in the subprime mortgage market, to borrow an analogy from Dr. Mark Smith. Speaking at a panel discussion on the future of employer health coverage, Dr. Smith presciently observed (in November 2006, months before the subprime mortgage meltdown began):

---

25 Evidence for this conclusion is provided by the recent experience with universal coverage in Massachusetts, where costs exceeded projections and the supply of primary care providers has been insufficient for the increase in the insured population (even though Massachusetts has the nation's third highest proportion of primary care physicians to the state population). Similar problems are anticipated when the national health reform legislation takes effect. See O'Reilly, K. Health reform's next challenge: Who will care for the newly insured? *American Medical News*, April 12, 2010, available at http://www.ama-assn.org/amednews/2010/04/12/prl10412.htm.

... no matter how much we tinker around with the insurance product, if in the end the care into which it buys you is unaffordable, it's like getting increasingly creative with your mortgage for a house you cannot afford. A lot of Americans over the next few years are going to be very sorry they did that . . . because they were trying to buy a financial instrument that would get them title to an underlying asset they could not afford. . .

To the extent that insurers and providers both see the problem of the uninsured as a revenue problem—which is to say, there are all these people out there who aren't part of our system, and we need to find a way to buy them into our system at more or less our system's price, at more or less our system's configuration, and more or less maintain the incomes of everybody in our system—that is a very different question from how can we make the underlying asset more affordable. . . .[26]

The underlying asset is delivery of medical care. Its affordability depends in large part on the behaviors of both providers and consumers. Their behaviors depend in large part on the system within which they function—on the infrastructure of standards and tools and processes for decision making, feedback and accountability. Transforming that infrastructure must be the foundation for health care reform.

Policymakers recognize that transformation requires more than technology. Accordingly, certification and "meaningful use" of electronic health records (EHRs) are required to receive subsidies to purchase EHRs under the 2009 economic stimulus legislation.[27] But the requirements for certification and meaningful use as currently conceived[28] are primitive. They fail to incorporate or even consider most elements of the problem-oriented medical record (POMR) standard (the subject of part VI), which became prominent four decades ago. Since that time, the quality of medical records has declined. Use of the POMR standard has receded, and the clinical purpose of the medical record has been compromised. The latter phenomenon was observed in 1992:

The medical record is already changing in subtle ways that few people are objecting to or even noticing. Much of the record now functions as an annotated bill prepared for third-party payers. This can have the chilling

---

26   http://healthaffairs.org/blog/2006/11/17/insurance-deconstructing-insurance.

27   See generally the "HITECH Act" provisions in Title IV of Division B of the American Recovery and Reinvestment Act of 2009, Pub. L. 111-5, 123 Stat. 115.

28   See generally the final regulations at 75 Fed. Reg. 44314 and 44590 (July 28, 2010) and part VI.B.

effect of making our patients appear sicker than they are, as physicians strive to add enough pathologies (and ICD-9 codes) to justify the hospital and physician services the patient is receiving. We need to think about ways to reclaim the chart for the patient.[29]

This corruption of medical records is now so entrenched that current observers see it as the norm, not as a decline from what medical records used to be. A July 2010 article states:

The old problem many physicians are trying to solve with an EHR is the efficient generation of a progress note—a document used to justify payment in a fee-for-service system, in which an office visit is the unit of value. ... [EHRs facilitate] more aggressive fee-for-service coding and more frequent use of higher-level primary care billing codes, both supported by more comprehensive documentation. ... However, primary care practice poses a different problem: managing the massive amount of information received about patients every day and using it quickly, efficiently, and safely to meet patients' needs.[30]

Failures of quality in medical records, paper and electronic, are a root cause of the health care system's failures of economy. The HITECH Act reforms effectively acknowledge this reality, but fail to remedy it (as we shall see in part VI.B below).

Health information technology has only recently become prominent in health care reform debates. The traditional focus of health care reform has instead been economic incentives. Yet, incentives are not the central problem. No arrangement of economic incentives is perfectly aligned with patient interests, especially within an out-of-control system (see part III.B below). Moreover, providers already have strong legal, professional and personal incentives, and to some extent economic incentives as well, to deliver cost-effective care. Consumers already have strong incentives to avoid the burdens and risks of unnecessary or ineffective care, regardless of who pays for it. Rather than incentives, the central problem, clearly illustrated by the case study in part II.A, is that providers and consumers too often are unable to act on incentives effectively.

This is not to deny the importance of economic incentives (which should at least not be aligned against patient interests). Nor is it to deny that incentives can be improved by shifting from managed care to well-designed consumer-

---

29   Donnelly, W, Brauner D. Editor's Correspondence: Why SOAP Is Good for the Medical Record?: Another View-Reply. *Arch Intern Med*, Dec. 1992; 152: 2511.

30   Baron R. "Meaningful Use of Health Information Technology Is Managing Information. *JAMA*, 304(1):89-90 (July 7, 2010). See also the discussion at notes 163-168 below.

driven care arrangements. Unlike managed care, the consumer-driven care concept recognizes the consumer's central role in the health care marketplace. But the consumer-driven concept is incomplete. Allying itself with the medical profession against third party payers, the consumer-driven care movement has turned backwards to traditional medical practice. Traditional practice, however, is provider-driven, in denial of the consumer's central role in medical decision making and execution. That central role was recognized decades ago in first developing the reforms advocated here.[31] The next section outlines how those reforms would complete the concept of consumer-driven care.

d. Consumer-driven spending and consumer-driven care

Two core elements of consumer-driven health plans—tax-sheltered spending accounts and high deductible insurance coverage—implicate health care spending. The theory is that consumer-driven spending arrangements shift some payment authority from third parties to consumers. This shift gives consumers some benefit from spending economically and increases consumer power over the provider reward system. But consumer-driven *spending* arrangements are not enough to bring about consumer-driven *care*.[32]

Consumer-driven care should be highly individualized care, driven by unique individual needs, not by the idiosyncrasies of providers or by the dictates of third party payers. Yet, the consumer-driven care movement has yet to define the clinical standards and tools and systems and processes needed for individualized medical problem solving.

Consider what happens when a physician first encounters a consumer with a medical problem for diagnosis or treatment. Were the encounter driven by the consumer's needs, the physician's initial data collection and analysis would not vary from one physician to another. Yet, initial data collection and analysis in fact vary enormously depending on which physician the consumer sees first. This variation at the front end of medical decision making is driven by provider idiosyncrasies, not individual consumer needs. Those individual needs continue to be neglected at the back end, when treatment decisions are made. At that stage, treatments are very often not individualized to the unique needs of each consumer. Instead, physicians fall back on limited personal knowledge, or

---

31 Weed, LL. *Medical Records, Medical Education and Patient Care* (1969), pp. 46, 48 ("In the last analysis, the patient with a chronic disease must in large part be his own physician ... patients are the largest untapped resource in medical care today").

32   This discussion is adapted from Weed L., Consumer Driven Spending or Consumer-Driven Care—Which Is It?, in "Exclusive Faculty Survey and White Papers on Improving Consumer-Driven Care," from the Second National Consumer-Driven Care Summit, Sep. 2007.

customary local practice, or one-size-fits-all dictates of third party payers, or the marketing messages of pharmaceutical and medical device manufacturers, or "evidence-based" standards derived from large population studies.

A true consumer-driven system would take precisely the opposite approach to decision making. The front end would not be variable but highly standardized. At the back end, decisions would become individualized.

At the front end, for both diagnostic and therapeutic decision making, the consumer and practitioner would begin by jointly following pre-defined, scientific standards (best practices) for initial investigation of the consumer's specific medical problem. Those standards would require detailed initial data collection. But this would involve nothing more than simple, quick, safe, and inexpensive findings from taking a history, performing a physical examination and doing basic lab tests, each designed in advance to elicit the data known to be most useful for analyzing the presenting problem. Software guidance tools would inform the consumer and practitioner what data are needed and what the findings mean (see part IV below).

This standardized collection of detailed initial data would reveal the medical uniqueness of different consumers who initially appear to present the same problem. Care would become individualized as it becomes obvious that different consumers labeled with the "same" presenting problem, or to whom a standard "evidence-based" treatment seems applicable, in fact may have very different medical needs, not to mention different preferences. Thus, in a truly consumer-driven environment, uniform "evidence-based medicine" would be seen as a crude substitute for individualized care. Consumers themselves would be seen as medical decision makers. Practitioners would be seen as experts in medical procedures, not as repositories of knowledge and not as decision making oracles. Medical "knowledge" itself would be seen as only a provisional approximation of medical reality for each individual consumer. That reality would be documented in highly structured electronic medical records. The records would be used to individualize each person's care over time in a highly organized and explicit manner (see part VI below). And feedback from those records could be harvested for continuously improving medical knowledge incorporated in software guidance tools (see the diagram at the end of part I).

This kind of infrastructure for individualized decision making, coupled with rigorous quality control of decision execution, would enable market forces to operate effectively. To paraphrase F. A. Hayek from another context, sound medical care requires practical knowledge that cannot be abstracted statistically from unique individual situations. That practical knowledge is only available to the person who is closest to the subject matter of the decision—and that person is the patient/consumer. But the patient/consumer cannot decide solely on the basis of his intimate but limited knowledge of his own medical situation. There still remains the problem of communicating to him such further information as he needs to fit his decision into patterns revealed by medical science.[33] Solving that problem requires information tools designed to integrate patient data with medical knowledge.

Without information tools of this kind, the quality and economics of care are disconnected from consumer needs. Rather than consumer-driven, the status quo is vendor-driven, by default. Reorienting this status quo to become truly consumer-driven requires subjecting vendors to basic standards of orderly problem solving . These are simple, common-sense standards of care that all consumers themselves can readily understand: systematic information gathering, problem definition, planning, follow-through, feedback and corrective action. At each step, provider inputs are explicitly defined and carefully controlled.

This kind of order and transparency has enabled the domains of science and commerce to develop and disseminate scientific knowledge and new technologies for the benefit of all, and to do so more reliably and productively than has ever occurred in the domain of medical practice.

In a truly consumer-driven system as just described, consumers are no longer passive beneficiaries of care delivered by autonomous physicians. Instead, consumers are active, informed users of an ordered, transparent system of care that they can trust. A system of that kind is incompatible with the traditional ideal of physician autonomy in the provider-driven model. Autonomy is a false ideal, one that leads physicians to resist necessary definition and control of their inputs to care.

Physician resistance in part reflects the self-protection of an entrenched profession facing little competition. But physician resistance also reflects a legitimate distrust of existing controls over medical practice. In the next part we examine an alternative—the concept of defined inputs to care—distinguishing this concept from controls over practice that physicians rightly resist.

---

33   F.A. Hayek, "The Use of Knowledge in Society," American Economic Review, XXXV, No. 4, Sep. 1945, pp. 519-30 at p. 18. As discussed further in Part V.B below, Hayek was not writing about medical care; his subject was the price system as a mechanism for communicating information.

III.
The Concept of Defined Inputs

He who would do good to another must do it in Minute Particulars.
General Good is the plea of the scoundrel, hypocrite, and flatterer;
For Art and Science cannot exist but in minutely organized Particulars

— *William Blake*[34]

A. The need for defined inputs

To some, any notion of defined or controlled inputs is anathema. The notion suggests conformity to external restrictions by *exclusion* of inputs—ignoring relevant information and suppressing clinical judgment. Indeed, this exclusion is evident in both the simplistic "cookbook medicine" of managed care guidelines and the more sophisticated "evidence-based medicine" of academia. To critics of those approaches, the notion of defined or controlled inputs sounds like a pseudo-scientific euphemism for compromising professional autonomy and the "art of medicine." From that perspective, health information technology threatens to become an insidious mechanism for imposing external control.

This skepticism reflects more than recent experience with managed care and evidence-based medicine. It reflects also a broader critique of formal, rule-based approaches to expert decision making in many fields. In medicine this critique has been directed at clinical protocols, statistical decision analysis and computer-based tools for decision making. As summarized in a study by Marc Berg, this critique idealizes the "art of medicine" and physician autonomy:

> Decision-analytic techniques ... are but poor representations of the complexities that go into real-time decision making. One cannot separate the decision from its context ... Such rigid, pre-determined schemes [as protocols] are said to threaten the physician's "art" by dehumanizing the practice of medicine and by reducing the physician to a "mindless cook" ... Moreover, such tools open the way for increased and uninformed controls by "outsiders." ... All in all, these critics argue, the tools' impoverished,

---

34   William Blake, "*The Holiness of Minute Particulars,*" *Jerusalem, ch. 3 (1820).*

codified versions of physicians' know-how do not do justice to the intricate, highly skillful nature of medical work. The idea of creating formal tools that make medical decisions is utterly mistaken. Every attempt to take practical control of the decision process out of the physician's hands is doomed to fail – and is dangerous.[35]

Physicians are right to condemn forms of control that involve exclusion of information and power over decision making. But physicians are in denial about the extent to which they themselves impose these forms of control on patients. Physicians are right to reject impoverished, cookbook medicine, but they are in denial of how impoverished is their own know-how. So too are they in denial when they view themselves as "highly skillful," because their levels of skill would be far greater within a disciplined system of care. Physicians are right that "one cannot separate the decision from its context," and they are right to reject "uninformed controls by 'outsiders.'" But they are in denial of how much they themselves are uninformed outsiders to patients' lives, outsiders whose exercise of control inevitably separates medical decision making from its context. And they are in denial of the need to submit to different forms of control over their own *inputs* to care—both decision making inputs and execution inputs.

Execution inputs were the primary focus of the Institute of Medicine's *To Err is Human.* That report highlighted the need to protect patient safety by exercising tight control over execution of medical procedures.[36] When we turn from execution to decision making, it is best to think in terms of not controlling but *defining* inputs, that is, making explicit the inputs that form the basis for decisions.

The basic inputs to decision making are (1) medical knowledge, (2) patient data and (3) the processing of that information. All three of those inputs are undefined and uncontrolled when they originate from the unaided minds of physicians. No one can know exactly *what* information physicians take into account, nor can we know *how* they take it into account, nor can we reliably improve the cognitive processes involved. All we know for certain is that medical decisions are enormously variable. The outcome is that patients have no assurance of reliable decision making, as the case study above illustrates all too clearly.

---

35   Berg M. *Rationalizing Medical Work.* Cambridge, MA: MIT Press, 1997 (p. 7).

36   Institute of Medicine, *To Err Is Human* (Washington: National Academy Press, 1999), p. 55 ("This report addresses primarily ... errors of execution, since they have their own epidemiology, causes and remedies that are different from errors of planning"), available at http://books. nap.edu/openbook.php?record_id=9728&page=55.

In contrast, a system of defined inputs means first that the knowledge and data taken into account, and the processing of that information, are explicitly defined. Second, it means exercising some degree of control over the manner in which the defined elements are combined. Defining inputs to decisions in this way does not dictate those decisions any more than defining the elements of writing (an alphabet and standards of spelling and grammar) dictates the content of writing.

The need for tight definition and control over inputs goes without saying when the inputs are drugs and medical devices. An elaborate regulatory scheme controls entry into the marketplace and ongoing manufacture of drugs and devices. Yet, nothing comparable exists for the most important medical devices of all—the minds and hands of physicians.[37] Graduate medical education, state law credentialing and board certification purport to regulate the entry of new physicians into the marketplace, while various *ad hoc* interventions (such as malpractice litigation and licensure board disciplinary proceedings) purport to regulate ongoing performance. Yet, no one trusts these forms of control. Epidemics of medical error, unnecessary care and irrational spending confirm that trust is not warranted. The reason is that existing regulation fails to define and control inputs to care comprehensively.

This means continually optimizing care at every step of decision making and execution. Optimizing care means not only enforcing high standards of care but also continuously incorporating feedback and new scientific advances. This continuous and comprehensive improvement entails a constant assault upon the status quo—upon the habits and roles and economic claims that take root from established practices. Trust will naturally arise when definition and appropriate

---

37   Indeed, physicians are legally permitted to prescribe drugs for unapproved, "off-label" uses, contradicting regulatory control over pharmaceutical companies, which are not authorized to market drugs for those uses. See Field R., *Health Care Regulation in America* (Oxford University Press, 2007), pp. 131-32 (characterizing this as "an anomaly of the American pharmaceutical regulatory scheme"). Some off-label prescribing might be justified if it took place within a system of defined inputs, where these prescribing decisions are made only when better alternatives for individual patients are shown not to be available and only when the meticulous, individualized outcome evaluations take place. But no such system exists for defining and improving the inputs to prescribing decisions. On the contrary, off-label prescribing is permitted on the basis of "supporting the ability of physicians to prescribe according to their best clinical judgment." Mello M. et al, Shifting Terrain in the Regulation of Off-Label Promotion of Pharmaceuticals, *New Eng. J Med.* 360:1557-1566 (April 9, 2009) (discussing regulation of covert promotional practices by pharmaceutical companies but not examining the basis of physician clinical judgment in off-label prescribing). In any event, off-label prescribing is only one of the problems in prescribing practices. See the discussion at note 142 below.

control are brought to the functioning of practitioners in all of its minute particulars. This requires standards, feedback, enforcement and improvement.

B. Modes of defining inputs

The first step is break down the innumerable particulars of medical practice into different categories of functioning. The two basic categories of functioning are decision making and execution of decisions. Decision making, in turn, is usefully conceived in two distinct stages: (1) assembling the informational *basis* for decisions to identify the available options with the pros and cons of each, and (2) choosing among the options in light of the evidence, judgment and personal values.[38] In the first stage, the information assembled should meet high standards of accuracy, completeness and objectivity. Those standards cannot be met as long as the unaided mind is the primary tool used to assemble the information. Tools external to the mind, and standards of care external to the personal habits and judgments of practitioners, are essential.

It is crucial to understand that these external tools and standards establish a *minimum* (albeit rigorous) level of performance. Individual freedom to *exceed* the minimum—to take into account information above and beyond that which is assembled externally—must be preserved. But no one should be free to fall short of the minimum by relying on inaccurate, incomplete or biased information.

Beyond external tools, external standards and individual freedom to exceed the minimum level of care, another element is crucial: a system of *feedback*. Corrective feedback enables response to variations from minimum standards. The personal judgments of individuals may be better or worse than knowledge captured with information tools, and new information from external sources must continuously be incorporated in the tools (recall the diagram at the end of part I). Feedback makes the occurrence and effects of variations transparent. Variations for the worse must then be systematically corrected, while variations for the better (proven innovations) must be systematically reproduced. Feedback loops should be built in throughout, so that tight control over cognitive inputs is maintained from the initial patient encounter to the final resolution of the patient's problem. In that way, continuous correction and improvement are enforceable as a natural byproduct of ongoing processes of care. Conceived in these terms, definition and control of inputs provide a foundation for evolutionary improvement in the *basis* for decision making, without interference in decision making itself.

---

38   Weed LL., Weed L. "Reengineering Medicine," *Federation Bulletin: The Journal of Medical Licensure and Discipline*, 1994; 81:147-83 (at p. 150), available at www.pkc.com/papers/reengineering.pdf.

As with decision making, control over execution inputs involves defining and disseminating high minimum standards of performance, obtaining feedback on actual performance, enforcing the standards and continuously improving them. For individual practitioners, control over inputs requires performance standards, not educational standards. Standards of performance involve periodic demonstrations of skill and correct technique in actually performing discrete medical procedures. For institutional providers, standards of performance (accreditation) must involve high standards of reliability for the myriad tools and systems and processes that institutions provide to support individual practitioners. And advances in technique and procedures must be rapidly incorporated in the standards to which individuals and institutions are held. These principles require transformation of medical education and credentialing, as discussed in part VIII.

This focus on inputs differs fundamentally from a focus on outcomes as the basis for quality improvement. That basic distinction has long been recognized in health policy discussions ("process" and "outcome" is the terminology ordinarily employed). A similar distinction—that between improving systems (inputs) and holding individuals accountable for errors (outcomes)—is now commonplace in discussions of patient safety and medical error. In that context, most now recognize that blaming individuals is ineffective at controlling the relevant inputs. As the Institute of Medicine has observed, "even apparently single events or errors are due most often to the convergence of multiple contributing factors. Blaming an individual does not change these factors and the same error is likely to recur."[39] Stated differently, holding an individual responsible for an adverse outcome does not change the multiple inputs leading to that outcome.

The patient safety movement has thus recognized that a key to preventing errors of execution is tight definition and control of inputs. Imposing liability or rearranging financial incentives are not enough. Definition and control are achieved by analyzing and improving each of the minute particulars of the process in question.

Nothing can remove the reality that "to err is human." Definition and control of inputs therefore must often take the form of bypassing ineradicable human limits. This often means changing the division of labor between man and machine. A simple example is the problem of illegible medication orders by physicians. The solution is not penmanship lessons but computerized order entry systems. Similarly, in the decision making arena, the solution for missed diagnoses and overlooked treatment options by physicians is not continuing education classes or malpractice suits. The solution is software tools. In these

---

39   *To Err Is Human,* note 36 above, p. 42..

examples, the technological solution is superior because it reduces dependence on idiosyncratic, uncontrollable human inputs.

Inputs must be defined and controlled comprehensively. Otherwise, one uncontrolled segment limits the range of safe choices available to patients. (Recall our analogy with the transportation system in part I, where we described how the auto transportation system is regulated and maintained comprehensively, so that drivers can choose their routes and destinations freely.) Moreover, comprehensiveness creates an environment of organized, continuous improvement, in two mutually reinforcing ways. First, both practitioners and patients are enabled to translate medical science into daily medical practice far more effectively than ever before. Second, the operational standards and tools needed for this change foster conditions of transparency, control, feedback and competition throughout the health care marketplace. Those marketplace conditions in turn foster an evolutionary process of natural selection by market forces. The absence of these operational and marketplace conditions is why failures of quality and economy in health care seem so intractable.

To further explain these concepts, it is useful to compare alternative approaches to quality control and improvement in medical practice. First, managed care organizations have used financial incentives to influence physician decision making. Second, attempts have been made to use clinical outcome comparisons as measures of quality (for example, randomized clinical trials, or hospital "report cards" based on risk-adjusted mortality rates for various procedures). Third, some organizations have taken a process-oriented approach—specifying a limited number of required inputs (e.g. immunizations for infants, use of beta blockers in cardiac care) as quality indicators. The specified inputs involve only a fraction of the inputs actually delivered by providers. Finally, the recent "HITECH Act" focused on electronic exchange of health information, without a corresponding focus on what physicians do with the information they exchange.

What these approaches have in common is that they avoid comprehensiveness. Substantial physician autonomy is thereby preserved. Physicians are left free to determine how to act on financial incentives or how to improve outcomes or how to select and process electronic information they send and receive. Often their provision of required inputs is scrutinized for whether it occurs, not for whether it is appropriate or complete for each individual patient. Most of the "minute particulars" of care are left hidden inside a black box.

These hands-off approaches to quality improvement have not worked and cannot work. The black box must be opened. Without standards and tools and systems and processes needed to define and control inputs comprehensively, disorder too often defeats the best efforts to improve medical outcomes and financial results. Incentives, for example, do nothing in themselves to overcome the conditions of complexity and information overload that make it difficult to identify the correct diagnosis or the most cost-effective treatment. Moreover, incentives inevitably have unintended consequences when applied to an out-of-control system of care. Any form of fee-for-service reimbursement tends to cause overuse of care, while any form of per capita reimbursement tends to cause underuse. Measuring performance in terms of outcomes creates an incentive to avoid difficult cases where favorable outcomes are hard to achieve. Measuring limited inputs as indicators of quality creates incentives for overuse of the measured inputs and underuse of everything else. All these alternatives leave patients at risk that providers will act on narrow reimbursement incentives at the expense of total quality and individual needs.

The notion of comprehensively defining and controlling inputs to care may seem utopian and naïve. Medical care does not take place in controlled environments. Unlike a scientific laboratory or a factory floor (environments where precisely defined and controlled inputs are expected), medical care is delivered in chaotic environments. Patients appear with multiple problems. Providers must take into account all those problems, they do not control when patient problems appear, they may not consider any one patient problem in isolation from others, they do not control most of the variables affecting the course of events, and they face scarcity of time and resources. Given those uncontrollable conditions, some may conclude that physicians must have the autonomy and authority to proceed according to their best judgment, without being subject to external controls. On this view, medicine is more art than science, and any notion of defining or controlling inputs destroys the "art of medicine."

Precisely the opposite is the case. The fact that medicine is practiced in uncontrolled environments only heightens the necessity for providers to bring their own inputs under control. In Blake's words, "Art and Science cannot exist but in minutely organized Particulars." Igor Stravinsky made a similar point about composing music: "A mode of composition that does not assign itself limits becomes pure fantasy. ... The creator's function is to sift the elements he receives, for human activity must impose limits on itself. The more art is controlled, limited, worked over, the more it is free."[40]

The underlying principle is that all complex activities, and the functioning of all complex systems, depend on limits and structure and form. If the pH of the human body changes a few tenths of a point or the body's temperature changes a

---

40 Stravinsky, I. *Poetics of Music in the Form of Six Lessons* (Cambridge: Harvard University Press, 1947), p. 63. The discussion here draws on *Knowledge Coupling*, p. 92, and *Medical Records, Medical Education and Patient Care*, pp. 12-13, 128-29 (see note 2 above).

few degrees, the human being will die. If the musicians in a symphony orchestra go "out of synch" by a single beat, great music is reduced to noise. In that sense, the "art of medicine" is too often missing from medical practice. To define and control inputs by practitioners is central to the art of medicine. Until the art of medicine is conceived in those terms, the benefits of medical science, and the enormous benefits that electronic information technology holds in store, will remain out of reach for many.

Powerful evidence of that reality can be found in the work of Dr. Peter Pronovost.[41] By enforcing use of simple checklists, he has achieved remarkable outcome improvements for execution of basic medical procedures such as central line insertions, use of ventilators and pain management. The power of simple checklists is essentially that they define and control practitioner inputs—inputs on which the outcomes of complex activities depend.

In the words of Dr. Atul Gawande, checklists "remind us of the minimum necessary steps and make them explicit. They not only offer the possibility of verification but also instill a kind of discipline of higher performance."[42] These seem like "ridiculously primitive insights," Dr. Gawande observes. It does not take an advanced degree "to figure out what anyone who has made a to-do list figured out ages ago."[43] Nevertheless, checklists remain an innovation in medical practice, not an accepted discipline.

Dr. Pronovost's work with checklists has focused on execution of medical procedures. In contrast, the work described below (see parts IV and VI) is focused on medical decision making. The standards and tools we describe can be viewed as a highly organized network of interactive checklists. They are designed to enable individualized medical decisions and continuous feedback—feedback during care for each patient, and feedback thereafter to improve the knowledge inputs to the relevant "checklists."

Some readers may argue that "evidence-based medicine" offers a way to bring decision making inputs under control. The reality, however, is that evidence-based medicine in its current form heads in the wrong direction.

---

41   See, e.g., Pronovost P, Needham D, Berenholtz S, et al. An intervention to decrease catheter-related bloodstream infections in the ICU. *N Engl J Med* 2006; 355:2725-32.

42   Gawande, A. *The Checklist Manifesto* (New York: Henry Holt & Co. 2009), p. 36. Dr. Gawande finds examples of the power of checklists not only in medicine but in other fields (large-scale construction projects, for example), where the problem of managing extraordinary complexity has been largely solved. The solutions, Dr. Gawande argues, involve various forms of checklists.

43   *Ibid.*, pp. 39-40.

C. Failings of "evidence-based medicine" as a mode of control over cognitive inputs

Evidence-based medicine is a response to the disorder that results from dependence on the unaided mind. Limiting the role of variable physician knowledge and judgments, evidence-based medicine emphasizes standardizing decisions based on randomized clinical trials and other generally accepted evidence. This standardization resembles industrial approaches to quality improvement. Industrial approaches seek to minimize variation by standardizing inputs.

In medicine, standardization is often essential to improving execution of decisions. Likewise, when the informational foundation for medical decisions is built (initial data collection), standardization is essential (see part IV.G.3). But after initial data collection, decisions must become individualized over time, that is, increasingly variable and differentiated as the patient's uniqueness emerges from detailed data.

Inputs to care are usefully conceived as a progression of small steps, forming a path over time. Many have observed that different providers follow different paths for patients labeled with the same disease condition. Those differing paths are frequently viewed as unjustified variations in care. To remedy this variation, evidence-based medicine determines in advance an optimal path for a given medical condition, and directs every patient labeled with that condition down that path. The chosen path is based on outcome evidence from large population studies of the disease condition in question. In those studies only a few paths are compared, only limited provider inputs are controlled, and only limited allowance is made for individual patient differences in comparing outcomes. On this basis, one of the paths under comparison is chosen as superior. Requiring providers and patients to follow the chosen path is believed to lead to outcomes superior *in the aggregate* to the outcomes of following the other few paths under comparison.

The relevant comparison, however, is not among a few paths chosen by researchers but rather among the countless paths that millions of informed patients would choose for themselves. If each patient makes informed choices along the way, and if each choice is skillfully executed, then the path chosen by each patient will be unique, and optimal for that patient. The optimal paths will reflect patients' individual characteristics, needs and preferences. That variation results in outcomes that, individually and collectively, are superior to the outcomes that those patients would experience if variation is eliminated so that they all follow the best path pre-determined by evidence-based medicine standards. Equally important, the variations arising from informed, defined individual choices provide fertile material for research. The generalizations of medical knowledge can be tested against each patient's unique, individual reality, as shown in structured medical records. Tracing the linkages between outcomes and each step along the individual paths chosen by patients will reveal new medical knowledge—knowledge of risks and benefits, dangers and safeguards, encountered at each step. Different patients taking the same step (for example, using a specific drug) might do so while following very different pathways (for example, they might have different combinations of medical problems and experience different outcomes and side effects). Accumulating detailed data about each step and its context for thousands of patients may yield new medical knowledge of greater precision and utility than ever before. (That knowledge can be harvested with institutional arrangements depicted in the diagram at the end of part I.)

The key is to equip patients and their practitioners with tools and systems for making informed choices and documenting every step over time. Favorable outcomes will be a byproduct if each step along the way is under control—that is, carefully chosen, executed, monitored and adjusted. "Carefully chosen" requires that the choice be informed by all factors relevant to the context, including factors revealed by other patients' similar situations and factors specific to that individual patient.

Evidence-based medicine postulates, in effect, that controlled individual choices by different patients labeled with the same disease will converge on one or a few optimal paths for that disease, leading to superior outcomes. We postulate the opposite. When inputs are optimized by careful attention to individual characteristics, needs and values over time, the optimal paths for different patients will soon diverge. Different patients, even though initially labeled with the same disease condition, must find their own ways to favorable outcomes. The reason is that evidence-based generalizations about disease conditions capture only a few elements common to many patients. Left out are countless individual differences among them that bear on optimal decision making for each.

The goal must be to recognize significant individual variations in maximum detail, while eliminating variations due to mere provider idiosyncrasies. Evidence-based medicine fails to accomplish either of those goals. These goals can be attained only by meticulous definition and control of inputs, from the very outset of care. That means defining a total system of care, assuring reliable execution by practitioners at every step within that system, and continuously improving the system itself by tracing connections between each step and clinical outcomes.

IV.
The Foundation: Coupling Patient Data With Medical Knowledge

A. Defining initial inputs as the foundation of care

For the want of a nail the shoe was lost, For the want of a shoe the horse was lost, For the want of a horse a rider was lost, For the want of a rider the battle was lost, For the want of a battle the kingdom was lost. And all for the want of a horse-shoe nail.

— *Benjamin Franklin*

Orderly problem solving begins with gathering relevant information. Relevance is a function of purpose. In medicine, information is gathered for three basic purposes: (1) maintaining wellness, (2) identifying medical problems at an early stage, and (3) solving identified problems. The output of initial information gathering for these purposes is a database for decision making. The database elements relevant to the first two purposes comprise the *screening database*. The database elements relevant to the third purpose comprise the *initial workup* of each problem identified by the screening database plus any additional problems identified by the patient and provider. (The initial workup is sometimes referred to as the "present illness.")

Gathering a database should involve (1) careful *selection* of data relevant to the three purposes just stated, and (2) accurate *analysis* of the data to determine implications for the patient. Both selection and analysis require matching data with medical knowledge. The results of the matching process need to be organized for problem solving purposes. This total process of matching general medical knowledge with patient-specific data and organizing the results we refer to as *knowledge coupling*. Regardless of whether it is carried out by the unaided mind, software tools or both, knowledge coupling is inherent in developing a database for decision making.

Knowledge coupling is employed not only for the initial database but also for defining problems, formulating diagnostic or treatment plans, evaluating the results of those plans and modifying the plans as needed, all of which involve matching medical knowledge with patient data. Knowledge coupling is thus fundamental to all of medical decision making. But its importance is greatest, and most amenable to improvement, when developing the initial database. Indeed, undefined, uncontrolled inputs to the initial database are a root cause of harm and waste in patient care.

The pivotal importance of the initial database should come as no surprise. Complex activities rest on a foundation laid by initial choices. Initial choices commit scarce time and resources to a chosen course of inquiry or action. Yet, initial choices are very often made without considering or comprehending relevant information. The best choice may thus be delayed, rejected or overlooked. Initial errors of this kind, like Franklin's missing horseshoe nail, trigger chain reactions that often cannot be stopped or even perceived until too late. Known as "cascade effects" when they occur at the biological level, these harmful chain reactions also occur at the organizational level. They are a recurrent phenomenon in clinical care at both levels.[44][45] And events at both levels often interact to increase the risk and degree of harm to the patient. Characteristic elements in these chain reactions include multiplying of disorganized data collection and risky medical interventions, delay of beneficial treatment, escalating complexity and increased likelihood of error as a result.

Because initial choices have such great significance, complex activities are usefully conceived as : (1) *threshold* processes where initial information is considered and initial decisions are made; (2) subsequent *follow-up* processes where decisions are executed, feedback is received and new decisions are made. The element of feedback further highlights the importance of threshold processes, because careful initial planning is often needed to establish feedback laps.

A clear example of the importance of threshold processes medicine is the case study in part II.A. Months of unnecessary care and avoidable suffering were set in motion when "classic manifestations" of the correct diagnosis went unrecognized in the initial workup. Other examples appear frequently in the media. Consider the following:

- A Pulitzer-prize winning *Wall Street Journal* article reports on "a deadly discrepancy between the available medical knowledge about aortic aneurysms and the ignorance of many front-line physicians." Headlined

---

44   Deyo R. Cascade Effects of Medical Technology. *Annu. Rev. Public Health* 2002. 23:23-44
45   Mold, JW, Stein JF. The cascade effect in the clinical care of patients. *New England Journal of Medicine*, 1986. 314:512-14.

"Medical Ignorance Contributes to Toll From Aortic Illness,"[46] the article explains that aortic disease "kills an estimated 25,000 Americans a year ... a larger toll than that of AIDS and most kinds of cancer." Yet, many physicians are not aware of the prevalence of aortic disease, its risk factors, its presenting signs and symptoms, and important diagnostic and therapeutic advances in caring for the disease. The article suggests that front-line physicians are to blame for their "ignorance." Yet, such blame misses the point, because ignorance is inevitable. The article suggests that a new medical specialty for aortic illness is needed, but that too misses the point, because the illness, and thus the need for the specialist, are difficult to recognize. The point is that an orderly, structured investigation is essential from the outset of care, because aortic illness is only one of hundreds of possible disease conditions suggested by its various presenting signs and symptoms. If those diagnostic possibilities are systematically investigated from the outset, then prompt diagnosis and treatment of the underlying disease (whether it turns out to be aortic illness or something else) become readily achievable in many cases. The difficulty is that all physicians inevitably will be ignorant of some of those diagnostic possibilities, their manifestations and their treatments. It is thus crucial to minimize dependence on the personal knowledge of physicians or any other practitioners. Only then does it become possible to optimize diagnostic workups of presenting signs and symptoms, whatever their cause. Seen in this light, the *Wall Street Journal* headline radically understates the tragedy the article describes. Rather than "Medical Ignorance Contributes to Toll From Aortic Illness," a more accurate headline would have been, "Medical Disorganization Multiplies Toll From All Illness." And rather than blaming "the ignorance of many front-line physicians," who deserve help rather than blame for being less than omniscient, it would be more accurate to blame the leaders behind the front lines, "the best and the brightest" who are positioned to transform the disorganization faced by all practitioners and patients.

- A 1998 ABC News report[47] described the case of a patient who experienced fatigue and joint pain, progressing to muscle pain, worse fatigue, disorientation and double vision. She "consulted more than 20 different doctors in search of an explanation," without success. Finally, she turned to

---

46   Helliker K, Burton T. Medical Ignorance Contributes to Toll From Aortic Illness. *Wall Street Journal.* Nov. 4, 2003, p. A1, available at http://www.pulitzer.org/year/2004/explanatory-reporting/works/story7.html.

47   http://www.pkc.com/videos.aspx. The software described is from PKC Corporation.

Dr. Charles Burger. He first had her spend "about 30 minutes completing a detailed computer-generated questionnaire that posed virtually every question that medical science suggests is relevant to her symptoms of fatigue—more than 550 questions in all." Dr. Burger's computer software then coupled the questionnaire responses with a database of possible diagnoses associated with the responses. The patient's signs and symptoms "turned out to be a nearly perfect match for 'hyperventilation syndrome,' a shallow-breathing disorder that can gradually change the body's chemistry." The patient learned corrective breathing techniques, with the outcome that her health is "steadily improving."

Such examples suggest that optimizing the initial workup could pay enormous dividends.

Optimizing the initial workup must begin with defining inputs to the process of coupling general knowledge with patient-specific data. This knowledge coupling process is employed for both components of the initial database—the screening database and initial workup of any identified medical problems. The following discussion is limited to the initial workup. In part VI.C.1 below we address the screening database.

The knowledge coupling function may be carried out by the unaided human mind, or with the aid of software tools. Because the unaided mind is so unreliable and so inefficient at knowledge coupling, software tools are essential. The question thus arises—which should be used first when conducting the initial workup? Should the practitioner first apply personal knowledge and judgment, and then use software tools to help with unresolved problems? Or should the practitioner first use software tools and then turn to personal knowledge and judgment?

A central theme of this book is that software tools should be employed first. Stated differently, human thought should supplement but not substitute for software tools when the knowledge coupling function is performed. This principle constitutes a new standard of care for medical practice. It is completely contrary to the basic premises of medical education and credentialing. To understand these points, we first need to examine the underlying logical structure of the initial workup, and then compare alternative approaches to conducting it.

B. The structure of the initial workup

We all know what happens when a physician first examines a new patient. The physician's clinical judgment largely determines what questions are asked about the patient's "chief complaint" and medical history, what points are checked in the physical examination and what laboratory tests are ordered. Similarly, the physician's judgment is the primary vehicle for analyzing the data collected. Then the physician judges what data and analysis to include in the medical record. Cognitive inputs to the initial workup are thus not predefined but determined during the patient encounter. Similarly, as to manual inputs when performing the physical examination, the quality of performance by physicians and other practitioners is not verified in advance. Practitioners vary considerably in the skill they bring to performing physical examinations, and they are rarely subject to corrective feedback on the quality of their performance. In short, the initial workup is unreliable at many levels.

Optimizing this initial workup requires breaking it down into three steps—choice, collection and analysis of patient data. Specifically:

1. *Choice*: Initial data must be chosen for its cost-effectiveness in identifying diagnostic or therapeutic options. This requires linking one datum—the patient's problem—with comprehensive medical knowledge about cost-effective initial data.

2. *Collection*: All the chosen data must be collected by conducting the patient/family history, the physical examination and laboratory tests without error or omission.

3. *Analysis*: Once collected, the chosen data must be linked with comprehensive medical knowledge to determine what those initial data mean.

Combining the initial data and knowledge inputs should yield the following outputs: a set of options (diagnostic or therapeutic) worth considering for the patient, plus, for each option, evidence (patient data) for and against the option, with proposals for additional data to collect or therapeutic measures to initiate. Equipped with this information, the patient and practitioner apply judgment and preferences to make an initial choice among the options identified.

This basic structure applies to both diagnosis and treatment decisions. That both types of decision have the same logical structure is not surprising. Organized problem solving of any kind involves processing information to identify options, plus evidence for and against each option. This information processing provides the *basis* for decisions. The decision is made when the patient or practitioner applies judgment to choose among the options identified, based on the evidence, in light of personal preferences and values. The objective quality of the decision, and its subjective acceptability to the patient, both depend on optimizing the *basis* for that decision.

Optimizing the basis for decisions cannot be accomplished with the unaided mind. Only electronic tools are effective at carrying out steps 1 and 3—choice and analysis of initial data. The mind can no more carry out those steps in real-world medical practice than the eye can perceive what a telescope reveals in outer space. This chasm between the mind's limited capacities and those of external information tools has pivotal importance.

C. Two contrasting approaches to the initial workup

Upon this gifted age, in its dark hour,
Rains from the sky a meteoric shower
Of facts…they lie unquestioned, uncombined.
Wisdom enough to leech us of our ill
Is daily spun, but there exists no loom
To weave it into fabric…

— *Edna St. Vincent Millay*[48]

The three steps of the initial workup as just described traditionally depend on the physician's personal knowledge and judgment. The physician chooses and collects (steps 1-2) very limited initial data for purposes of quickly formulating initial conclusions or hypotheses (step 3). Applying clinical judgment throughout, the physician is highly selective with the first two steps, proceeding to the third step as soon as possible. No two physicians, given the same patient, get the same information or reach the same conclusions. Some physicians go straight to the "present illness" or "chief complaint"; others begin with a screening data base or "systems review." In either case, physicians use their own judgment in selecting data and deciding what the data mean. If the first iteration of this sequence is not successful, the physician keeps repeating the sequence with new data. This can be termed a *judgmental* approach, because it relies so heavily on the trained physician's sophisticated clinical judgment in choice and analysis of initial data. Its reliance on personal judgment means that this approach is not easily analyzed or improved.

A contrasting approach begins with defining a detailed, standardized database for a given diagnostic or management problem (step 1), taking all medical specialties into account, based on research of the medical literature. Constructed *before* any patient encounter, this database is entered into software designed to

---

48   Millay, E. Upon this age, that never speaks its mind. In: *Collected Sonnets*. New York: Harper & Row, York, 1988. p. 140.

be used *during* the patient encounter. In step 2, the patient and practitioner use the software as guidance for collecting all of the defined data for the given problem, whether or not the practitioner judges the data to be useful for an individual patient. In step 3, the software automatically links all of the data with comprehensive medical knowledge about the significance of the data points and their interrelationships. This linkage is a simple process of association, readily accomplished with software tools and without reliance on the practitioner's knowledge or judgment (see the chest pain example on pp. 1-2 above).

This alternative to the judgmental approach we term a *combinatorial* approach.[49] It uses computer software to combine data with knowledge, thus identifying medically significant combinations of data points. The combinatorial approach contrasts with the judgmental approach not only in its reliance on an external tool to determine decision making inputs, but also in the nature of these inputs:

- The level of detail, in both the data collected and knowledge taken into account, are much greater with the combinatorial approach.

- This detailed information is gathered and presented up front and all at once, rather than in a gradual, piecemeal fashion.

- Inputs are highly standardized (the data collection and identification of linkages to medical knowledge are determined uniformly, regardless of which provider the patient sees), unlike the highly variable inputs of the judgmental approach, where inputs depend on the practitioner's personal knowledge, experience, specialty orientation, reimbursement expectations, time constraints and other factors.

Driven by an external tool, the combinatorial approach immediately brings to bear the best current expertise, accumulated from the experiences of countless patients and practitioners over time, filtered through peer-reviewed medical literature. This distilled expertise establishes a minimum standard for the information taken into account, but not a limit on that information. Practitioners and patients are free to supplement the defined initial workup

---

49 "Combinatorial" simply means relating to or involving combinations. We use the term as a shorthand for the general concept of systematically working through numerous possible combinations of a finite set of elements. A combinatorial approach differs from an algorithmic approach, which involves following a sequence of instructions such as "if you see X, then do Y." It also differs from a probabilistic approach, which involves ranking options by their assumed probability. When applied in medical contexts, both algorithmic and probabilistic approaches are fraught with risk, because they operate to exclude potentially relevant possibilities from consideration. See generally the remainder of this part IV, part VII below, and *Knowledge Coupling*, note 2 above, pp. 38-40, 53-54.

with any additional data they judge useful, and are free to make their own connections between the patient data and medical knowledge in addition to the connections identified by the software. In contrast, the judgmental approach limits the initial workup to the data and connections suggested by the personal judgment of whatever practitioners happen to be available to the patient, with no assurance of satisfying minimum standards of completeness or accuracy.

The judgmental and combinatorial approaches contrast in terms of not only their inputs but their outputs. Specifically:

- The output of a combinatorial approach is not a clinical decision, but merely the informational *basis* for a decision: a set of options with patient-specific evidence for and against each option. The initial options and evidence are generated by the software tool , not by the physician's judgment. The decision to be made based on this output is left to the patient and practitioner. In contrast, the output of a judgmental approach naturally takes the form of the physician's recommendations plus a selective presentation of options and evidence, generated by exercise of the physician's clinical judgment.

- The combinatorial approach automatically generates complete documentation, which is available over time to the patient, multiple practitioners, and clinical researchers (see the diagram in part I). This documentation includes positive, negative and uncertain responses (whether or not the practitioner judges them to be significant). In contrast, typical physician notes are incomplete and ambiguous as to whether an unmentioned finding was found to be negative or uncertain or was never checked at all.

The judgmental approach, not the combinatorial approach, is the accepted standard of care in medicine. For example, standard coding guidance states that the physician "uses the presenting illness as a guiding factor and his or her clinical judgment about the patient's condition to determine the extent of" the history and physical examination.[50]

The judgmental approach is the accepted standard not only in routine primary care but also in advanced specialty practice. This conclusion might seem surprising because specialists frequently pursue detailed data collection, which is characteristic of the combinatorial approach. Such investigation, however, usually occurs *after* the initial workup, and after a crucial threshold judgment

---

50   Center for Medicare and Medicaid Services, Evaluation and Management Services Guide (Rev. July 2007), pp. 12-13, at http://www.cms.hhs.gov/MLNProducts/Downloads/eval_mgmt_serv_guide.pdf.

is made—the judgment of which specialist should be consulted first. Different primary care physicians or other gatekeepers vary in their judgments selecting the specialist, and physicians in different specialties vary enormously in how they approach a given patient problem (not to mention the variation that exists even among physicians within the same specialty). In contrast, the tool-driven combinatorial approach takes into account data and knowledge from all potentially relevant medical specialties at the outset of care, before any physicians exercise judgment. This deferral of judgment is critical, because patients often have multiple problems, and because even a single problem often implicates multiple body systems, each with its own medical specialty.

To summarize, the combinatorial and judgmental approaches are founded on incompatible premises:

- The basic premise of the judgmental approach is that firsthand clinical judgments of highly trained physicians interacting with patients should govern the initial workup. Physician judgments should not be compromised by second-hand, abstract, "evidence-based" generalities incorporated in clinical guidelines or software tools. Those external tools may have some utility as references to consult, but physicians should primarily rely on their own clinical judgment to determine the contents, and assess the results, of each initial workup for each unique patient.

- In contrast, the basic premise of the combinatorial approach is that detailed initial data for a given medical problem should be defined in advance and collected without fail for each patient presenting that problem. For this to happen, software tools, not clinical judgment during the encounter, should govern collection and analysis of the data. Ongoing clinical judgments of physicians may have some utility as a *supplement* to the combinatorial minimum standard, but should not be permitted to lower that standard.

D. The basis for choosing between the two approaches

Given these contrasting approaches to the initial workup, on what basis should we choose between them? Clinical trials do not provide a sound basis for choice, as discussed below and in Appendix A. Rather than attempting clinical trials, we should choose the approach to the initial workup that best contributes to building a total system of care.

To understand what we mean by a system of care, recall Parts I-III above, where, respectively, we analogized the transportation system, analyzed a case study in the *lack* of a system for the initial workup, and explained why a system requires defined inputs. Inputs are defined by the system's rules, not by the judgments and habits of practitioners. This concept of a system is familiar in many areas where we expect individuals to submit to predefined, externally imposed rules. In athletics, for example, the players are not free to define the rules during the game. In the economy, business executives are not free to ignore accounting rules. In law and politics, we speak of "the rule of law" and "a government of laws, not a government of men," meaning that individuals are not free to ignore rules defined by the legal system.

In addition to defining rules, a system integrates those rules into a transparent whole, understandable to the participants governed by it, giving them a framework for pursuing multiple interrelated purposes. A system of this kind avoids highly complex rules and does not involve centralized, top-down controls (points we discuss further in part V.B below). Rather, it involves rules simple enough to be applied by all participants in the system. Thus, for example, a system of writing involves a simple alphabet and spelling rules, which individuals can use in countless ways for their own communicative purposes. Similarly, a health care system should involve simple rules that patients and practitioners can apply to countless, unique individual needs.

To define the simple rules for a health care system, some guiding principles must be followed. Underlying these principles is *accountability*: practitioners should be accountable for performing roles defined by the system, patients should be accountable for their own behaviors, the system itself should be accountable for medical outcomes attributable to the system's functioning—but no one should be held accountable for unattainable performance or uncontrollable outcomes.

Drawing on our discussion of defined inputs in part III, we can state the guiding principles for building an accountable system of medical care as follows:

- The system must define its goals and the rules for achieving those goals.

    o The rules must be comprehensive, not selective.

    o The rules must be attainable, not merely aspirational.

    o The rules must define the tools, processes, and standards of care needed to follow them.

    o The rules must define roles for all practitioners

    o Practitioner roles must be integrated, so that coordinated care results from practitioners' performing their defined roles.

- Individuals must be accountable for performance within the system's rules.

    o Defined practitioner roles must be specific standards for performing discrete medical procedures.

o   The standards must be set at a high, but attainable level.

o   Credentials to practice must be based not on educational preparation but on actual performance of defined roles, demonstrated periodically.

o   Practitioners must be held accountable for satisfying high standards of performance in their defined roles, not for the outcomes of care.

o   Patients must be held accountable for their own health behaviors.

- The system itself must be accountable for outcomes within its control.

o   The system must be able to distinguish between outcomes that are traceable to system inputs (e.g., medical procedures performed by practitioners or knowledge inputs from information tools) and outcomes that are traceable to factors outside of the system's control (e.g. patient behaviors, incurable disease, the social and physical environment).

o   System inputs that contribute to unfavorable outcomes must be continuously corrected and improved.

A health care system of this kind makes possible reliability, transparency, feedback and improvement. Building a health care system with these characteristics is incompatible with the judgmental approach to the initial workup. A system requires a foundation that only the combinatorial approach can establish.

The remainder of this part IV applies these principles in explaining the combinatorial approach to the initial workup and comparing the judgmental approach. The following points will serve to introduce that discussion and clarify these principles:

- The goal for the initial workup must be to collect and process the data needed for identifying all of the patient's current and foreseeable medical problems, to the extent justified by the costs and benefits involved. Defining the goal in these terms leads naturally to clear rules for the content of the initial workup.

- The goal just stated for the initial workup requires that its content be comprehensive and standardized. This is only attainable with a combinatorial approach using external information tools. The system must therefore equip practitioners with the necessary tools. Absent those tools, practitioners cannot be held accountable for overlooking needed data or implications of the data obtained.

- The rule that the data should be standardized means that practitioners should not have discretion to judge on a case-by-case basis which initial data are useful.

- The rule that data must be comprehensive means that it should enable a complete medical assessment, without being limited to the patient's chief complaint or the practitioner's specialty. But comprehensive does not mean exhaustive. The initial workup should include only data that are useful and cost-effective for identifying and initially analyzing patient problems.

- The initial workup should exclude data that in theory might be useful for initial problem identification and analysis but in practice involve procedures that are too costly, too risky, too painful, too uncertain or insufficiently beneficial to justify routine use at the outset of care. Examples are expensive imaging and invasive tests.

- Selected process or outcome measures of quality are no substitute for comprehensively defining a system of care. Merely selecting a limited range of process or outcome measures as *indicators* of overall quality, in the hope that unmeasured elements will correlate with those indicators, is unacceptable. That limited approach gives practitioners an incentive to conform to measured indicators while otherwise reverting to their usual discretionary judgments.

- Enforcing that combinatorial approach creates order and transparency in detailed patient data. Those data provide a foundation for tracing the connections between patient outcomes and system inputs.

- Order and transparency in detailed data also make it possible to search that data for new patterns and new connections with scientific research, thereby changing current disease profiles, concepts and classifications. It will become possible to revisit both archaic and modern notions of disease, ranging from Hippocrates, who saw disease as pervading the entire body, to Morgagni, whose anatomical studies in the 18th century linked specific diseases to particular organs, to modern genetics, which links diseases to genetic variations.

In short, a system of care protects against the variable habits, abilities and judgments of autonomous practitioners. Rather than accepting clinical judgment, a system minimizes the need for it. Rather than granting professional autonomy, a system defines professional roles. Rather than perpetuating historic roles, a system redefines those roles, optimizing the division of labor among practitioners, patients, and external tools.[51]

None of this is possible using a judgmental approach to the initial workup. Nevertheless, some readers may believe that the combinatorial approach should be tested against the judgmental approach using randomized clinical trials (RCTs). (Indeed, such comparisons have been attempted, as we discuss in Appendix A.) This view perhaps reflects beliefs that unintended consequences result when we disrupt the status quo, that the burden of proof should rest on those who would do so, and that RCTs are an effective way to carry that burden of proof.

In medicine, these beliefs do not withstand analysis. The status quo is itself riddled with unintended consequences. The burden of proof should rest on those who would perpetuate the harmful status quo, not on those who offer rational change. Moreover, we can compare the status quo with proposed changes by conducting thought experiments, with simple logic and existing evidence. Existing evidence offers no support for the judgmental approach. The human mind's inability to cope with the complexity of medical practice has been apparent for a century or more. This gap has only widened with ever-increasing scientific knowledge. The power of software tools to cope with complex information has already been demonstrated in many contexts, including medicine.

For these reasons, spending scarce time and resources on RCTs would be pointless. The point is to build and continuously improve a defined system of care, not to compare it with the failed status quo.

Even if that comparison were thought useful, RCTs comparing the combinatorial and judgmental approaches cannot be conducted with scientific rigor. The judgmental approach lacks the order and transparency that would be needed for valid comparison. This is especially true for comparisons based on outcomes. Outcomes, whether medical or economic, depend on countless variables in patients, providers, and their surroundings. Most of those variables cannot be held constant or rigorously accounted for. That is why, as Don Berwick has observed, the "typical conclusion" from traditional clinical trials is "the assertion either that nothing works or that the results are inconsistent and that more research is needed." Writing about inconclusive results in RCTs for rapid clinical response team systems, Dr. Berwick explains:

---

51 Weed LL, "Physicians of the Future," *New England Journal of Medicine*, 304: 903-907, April 9, 1981.

The introduction of rapid response systems in hospitals is a complex, multicomponent intervention—essentially a process of social change. The effectiveness of these systems is sensitive to an array of influences: leadership, changing environments, details of implementation, organizational history, and much more. In such complex terrain, the RCT is an impoverished way to learn."[52]

Dr. Berwick goes on to criticize the traditional RCT model as focusing too single-mindedly on the question of "'whether a [social] program works at the expense of knowing why it works.'"[53] In its pursuit of "generalizable knowledge," the traditional model depends on "removing most of the local details about 'how' something works and about the 'what' of contexts." He also criticizes attempts to eliminate bias by insisting on third party evaluators. "Almost always, the individuals who are making changes in care systems know more about mechanisms and contexts than third party evaluators can learn with randomized trials." Rather than attempting third party evaluation, the "better plan is to *equip the workforce to study the effects of their efforts, actively and objectively, as part of daily work*" (emphasis added). That is precisely what is accomplished with the tool-driven, combinatorial approach.

This is not to deny the need to guard against the risks inherent in disrupting the status quo. The status quo includes many unseen adaptations developed by individuals to protect against its failings. Changes to the status quo must therefore be introduced with care, ensuring that everyone understands why the status quo is unacceptable and how the change will improve it. RCTs distract from that effort.

Many argue for an evidence-based approach to innovation, correctly pointing out that safety and quality practices that seem promising may turn out to be ineffective, too costly or even harmful. Robert Wachter (see note 52 above) gives the example of universal screening for methicillin-resistant staph aureus (MRSA) infections, an approach that may be inferior to strictly enforcing simple hand hygiene practices. But he acknowledges that those simple practices do not need to be justified by RCTs. The combinatorial approach to the initial workup is no less basic and no less justified than hand hygiene. Our minds require cleansing no less than our hands when used in patient care.

52   Berwick D. The Science of Improvement. *JAMA*, 299:10; 1182-1183 (Mar. 12, 2008). Compare Wachter R., The Great Quality Debate: Berwick's Plea for Action vs. Evidence-based Medicine (Mar. 17, 2008), http://community.the-hospitalist.org/blogs/wachters_world/archive/2008/03/17/this-week-s-jama-berwick-s-plea-for-action-confronts-evidence-based-medicine.aspx.

53   Berwick, note 52, quoting Pawson R., Tilley N. *Realistic Evaluation*. London: Sage Publications, Ltd. 1997.

Moreover, any attempt to use RCTs to comparing the combinatorial and judgmental approaches is destined to become bogged down in complexity and controversy. This is especially true when comparison is based on outcomes. The effects of the countless variables relevant to outcomes cannot realistically be accounted for when comparing the two approaches. The combinatorial approach is transparent—it enables detailed accounting of initial data and knowledge inputs, and it is designed to be used in conjunction with highly structured, problem-oriented medical records that bring similar order and transparency to follow-up processes of care. In contrast, the judgmental approach is opaque— inputs are hidden inside the physician's mind—and it is used in conjunction with haphazard record-keeping practices that further undermine order and transparency. This means that the judgmental approach does not permit rigorous analysis of patient characteristics, provider actions, ultimate outcomes and the connections among those variables. Without that analysis, comparison between the two approaches would inevitably be disputed, and those disputes could not be resolved from the data. Thus, the security blanket of definitive outcome comparisons is simply not available.

These conclusions should not be surprising. Recall the concept with which this document began. We began by asserting the need for a secure *foundation* for care. With buildings, the value of a secure foundation is obvious, even though it gives no assurance that the rest of the building is well designed, constructed or maintained. That lack of assurance does not make the foundation any less important. On the contrary, if the foundation is not secure, then the rest of the building, no matter how well designed, constructed or maintained, is untrustworthy. And in medicine, the complex processes of patient care are untrustworthy if relevant, available information is not taken into account at the outset of care.

E. Objections to the combinatorial approach

Physicians naturally view the judgmental approach, and the elaborate training needed for the unaided mind to apply it, as inherent in scientifically advanced medical care. By comparison, a tool-driven, combinatorial approach seems to impose both crude standardization and excessive detail—"cookbook medicine" taken to a compulsive extreme. These general reactions can be broken down into the following five specific points:

- A combinatorial approach seems prohibitively time-consuming and expensive to physicians, because the knowledge coupling software employed in the combinatorial approach requires routinely collecting data (step 2 of the initial workup) in greater detail than is customary or feasible when rapid throughput of patients is an economic necessity.

- Whatever its feasibility, detailed data collection at the outset of care seems unproductive to physicians. On this view, detailed initial data collection results from premature concern with unlikely possibilities (rare diagnoses, non-standard treatments). Limited time and resources logically should be directed first at the most common and likely possibilities. Knowledgeable physicians can frequently avoid the time and expense of detailed data collection, as illustrated by the physician who correctly diagnosed the Addison's disease case based on very limited initial data (see part II.A.2 above).

- Physicians view the *standardized* data collection involved in a combinatorial approach as mere cook-book medicine. Every patient and every practice setting are different. Selecting which data are clinically useful for each patient in any particular setting (step 1 of the initial workup) must be judged by the physician during each patient encounter.

- Physicians object that the combinatorial approach harms the doctor-patient relationship. Because the patient interacts initially more with a computer and non-physician personnel than with the physician, the combinatorial approach gives the physician less opportunity to observe the patient's condition firsthand and establish a personal relationship.

- Physicians believe that mere information processing by external software tools can never substitute for their informed clinical judgment. Like experts in other advanced fields of knowledge, physicians solve complex problems by applying first principles to the specifics of the situation in a subtle and discriminating manner that no software can replicate. Nor can software replicate physicians' intuitive, instinctive judgments arising from their personal interactions with patients.

Much of the above critique originates in the culture of graduate medical education. That culture teaches reliance on personal intellect. Medical students are first selected for academic proficiency. Then they learn that they must acquire vast medical knowledge. Then they learn to rely heavily on their own intellectual powers when applying that knowledge to detailed patient data. Then they submit to knowledge-based standards for licensure and board certification. Their ordeal indoctrinates physicians with faith in the efficacy of intellect. Reinforcing this faith are the high compensation and status physicians receive for exercising their clinical judgment. Moreover, they are legally insulated from competition by other practitioners who might deliver superior care by avoiding faith in personal intellect.

Not only physicians but their patients acquire this faith. We are all socialized to believe, as the great clinician Herman Blumgart once wrote, that "application of knowledge at the bedside is largely the function of the sagacity inherent in or personally developed by the individual physician."[54] This ideal of personal sagacity was described by Sherwin Nuland. Recall his description of how physicians seek to solve "The Riddle," to determine the diagnosis and design a cure from their own understanding of pathophysiology. "Solving The Riddle ... is every doctor's measure of his own abilities; it is the most important ingredient in his professional self-image. ... Our most rewarding moments of healing derive not from the works of our hearts but from those of our intellects."[55]

Yet, the works of our intellects cannot be trusted. Those rewarding moments when our intellects solve The Riddle for some patients are inseparable from terrible moments when our intellects fall short for others. And the problem is not just fallibility. The problem is also that the best intellects can serve only a few. One physician's solution of The Riddle for one patient provides no foundation for improving the care of all patients by all practitioners. Those realities are the Achilles heel of the judgmental approach to the initial workup. A commitment to overcome those realities leads inevitably to the combinatorial approach, implemented with external information tools designed to make it practical.

F. A software implementation of the combinatorial approach

... a whole calling may have unduly lagged in the adoption of new and available devices. It may never set its own tests. There are precautions so imperative that even their universal disregard will not excuse their omission.

—Judge Learned Hand[56]

Physicians vary in their innate and acquired intellectual abilities. Moreover, even the most gifted and well-schooled intellects are not reliable when processing large amounts of information on the fly. This is precisely what steps 1 and 3 of the initial workup require (recall the three steps—choice, collection and analysis of patient data–from Part IV.B). This is where medicine most needs a new division of intellectual labor—a division between electronic tools that

---

54   Blumgart H., "Medicine: The Art and the Science," *Hippocrates Revisited*, R. Bulger ed. (New York: MEDCOM Press, 1973), p. 34.

55   Nuland, S. *How We Die*, note 17 above.

56   *The T. J. Hooper*, 60 F.2d 737, 740 (2d Cir. 1932).

process information, and users who, based on that information and personal values, apply judgment to arrive at decisions.

This division of labor exploits the fact that human judgment becomes increasingly accurate, efficient and powerful when it receives relevant information and is equipped to take that information into account— provided, however, that the information is specifically relevant to the problem at hand and not so voluminous or disorganized as to escape comprehension. The proviso is critical. An overload of extraneous or disorganized information brings back the very cognitive weaknesses to avoid.[57] Yet, medical education and credentialing pretend these cognitive weaknesses do not exist.

The culture of medicine must drop the pretense and instead enforce the consistent use of external information tools. Physician experts tend to resist this, because the tools expose their weaknesses and reveal how little they have to offer beyond information processing (see part IV.G.5 for further discussion).

To understand what the tools accomplish, we need to identify three distinct functions that information technology may perform:

1. storage and retrieval of general knowledge (e.g., Internet access to medical texts);

2. storage, retrieval and transmission of patient data (e.g., electronic medical records, telemedicine, health information exchange networks); and

3. linkage of patient-specific data with general knowledge for decision making purposes (e.g., computerized prescription order-entry systems that use patient data inputs to provide individualized guidance on medication selection and dosing, or the knowledge coupling software discussed below).

The difficulty of each of these three functions has been escalating dramatically for a century, with the extraordinary growth of medical knowledge and corresponding patient data. Performance of the first function has successfully kept pace with this growth, thanks to electronic tools for knowledge storage and retrieval. Performance of the second function, however, has not kept pace, in part because of lack of interoperability among different technologies, and in part because of the disorganized state of medical records as discussed in part VI

---

57 "The problem of information overflow represents a fundamental informatics problem, and will require some redesign of current clinical systems. It should be possible to 'strain out' much of the extraneous information, while highlighting the few items that are truly need to be addressed soon." Bates D. Getting in Step: Electronic Health Records and Their Role in Care Coordination. *J Gen Intern Med* 25(3):174–6 (2010).

below. Here, our concern is the third function – linking data with knowledge. Paradoxically, improvement in the first two functions makes this third function all the more difficult. That is, new tools for the first two functions increase the volume of accessible knowledge and data to combine and comprehend

That third function is at stake in steps 1 and 3 of the initial workup. Recall that step 1 involves linking one datum – the patient's problem – with comprehensive medical knowledge about the additional data needed to investigate that problem. Once collected (step 2), the chosen data must be linked with all relevant knowledge (step 3) in order to "connect the dots"—to comprehend the pieces of data that turn out to be useful, while filtering out extraneous data. The unaided human mind cannot perform this linkage function reliably or efficiently. The difficulty is not just that the volume of medical knowledge exceeds what anyone can learn. (That problem diminishes with tools for efficient knowledge retrieval.) The deeper problem is that no one is able to link complex knowledge reliably with detailed patient data, especially when operating under real-world time constraints.

This is a familiar phenomenon. It occurred, for example, in the Addison's disease case described in part II.A. The inherent intellectual difficulty is often exacerbated by situation-specific or provider-specific constraints. A doctor may be so busy and distracted, or so fixated on possibilities within his specialty, that he fails to consider or follow through on possibilities that another physician might pursue immediately. Moreover, existing knowledge is imperfect. Actual patients often do not fit neatly into the patterns that education and experience lead physicians to expect (we will return to this crucial point in part VII). Every patient is unique in the combination of those characteristics and circumstances that bear on solving the patient's problem. Thus, the subset of data and knowledge that turn out to be useful differs for every patient, even patients labeled with the same disease. And that subset cuts across specialty boundaries. Medical specialties thus artificially restrict analysis. For these reasons, no one can know in advance the unique subset of data and knowledge that will prove to be relevant to each patient's needs.

One context in which the mind's limitations have become especially obvious is medication ordering in hospitals. In that context, most observers now recognize that judgmental and manual processes are no substitute for computerized prescription order entry (CPOE) systems. More than two decades of studies have documented compelling quality and cost improvements at institutions that enforce use of well-designed systems. If this is true for the limited function of medication ordering, then it should come as no surprise to find that electronic tools are essential in any setting that requires linkage of patient data with medical knowledge—*especially* the initial workup, the foundation for everything that follows, the point of maximum uncertainty, where the need for raw information processing is greatest.

Electronic tools should filter and organize all information potentially relevant to the problem at hand for the purpose of "connecting the dots" among the limited items of information actually relevant to the individual patient. Recall the chest pain example from pp. 1-2. Another example is described by the *Wall Street Journal* article on aortic aneurysms, discussed in part IV.A above. Another example is diagnosis of hypertension. Scores of possible causes (and other diagnostic associations) are usefully taken into account for safe and cost-effective diagnosis of the cause of hypertension. These diagnostic possibilities implicate numerous medical specialties. Cost-effectively identifying which of the diagnostic possibilities are relevant to an individual patient requires checking for the presence or absence of hundreds of distinct clinical findings from history, physical and laboratory data. Yet, most physicians consider only a fraction of all this information when conducting initial workups of hypertension.

Another especially important example is management of diabetes. Again, the medical literature shows that managing diabetes requires taking into account scores of different therapeutic options. Identifying the options relevant to an individual patient and initially assessing the pros and cons of the relevant options involves making hundreds of distinct findings at the outset of care. Again, most physicians consider only a fraction of all this information during initial workups of diabetic patients.[58]

Once made, all of the initial findings are coupled with a database of medical knowledge built into the knowledge coupling software. The software's output is a list of diagnostic or therapeutic possibilities (i.e. possibilities for which at least one expected finding appears in the patient), plus the evidence for and against each possibility (i.e. the expected findings that are present and those that are not present). The output also includes comments on findings and options for which further explanation is useful, and supporting citations to the medical literature. The software thus links data with general knowledge, filters out information not potentially relevant to the patient and organizes the rest, arranging it by the option to which the information relates. Complex information is presented in a

---

58   The examples given are based on searching the medical literature for purposes of building the knowledge coupling tools described here. As discussed below, the tools must enable the practitioner and patient to take into account the full range of possible causes and their interactions.

way that is maximally useful for solving the problem at hand. This total process is termed "problem-knowledge coupling."

The coupling process can be conceived as navigating through three concentric circles of knowledge and corresponding patient data. These three circles encompass diagnostic or therapeutic options for the individual patient, as shown below.

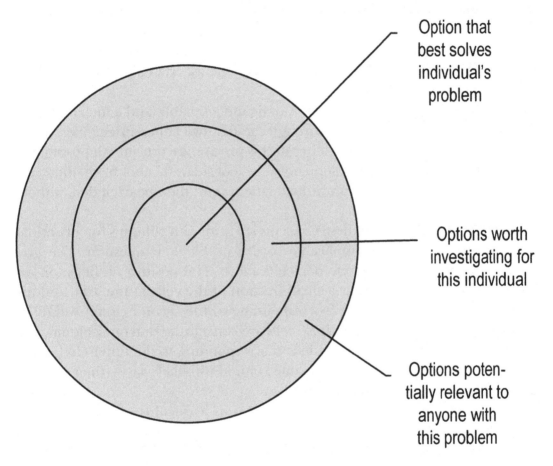

Option that best solves individual's problem

Options worth investigating for this individual

Options potentially relevant to anyone with this problem

The outer circle consists of all known options that are potentially relevant to the problem in question, plus, for each option, medical knowledge about the most useful initial data to collect for purposes of determining which options are worth investigating. This outer circle is completely standardized. The same data should be collected uniformly for all patients with the same presenting problem.

The middle circle is the subset of options, with corresponding knowledge and data, that are worth considering for an individual patient, based on data suggested by the outer circle and collected for that patient. The options worth considering are options for which at least one positive finding is made in that patient. Unlike the outer circle, the information in the middle circle is not standardized; it varies among different patients with the same presenting problem. The initial consideration of these options is simply comparing them to determine if one option stands out as the solution to the patient's problem, or, if not, which options are worth further investigation.

The inner circle is the option ultimately chosen as the best solution for the patient's problem. In some cases, the initial workup will be sufficient to locate this inner circle; in other cases, further investigation will be needed before a solution can be identified. In cases of genuine uncertainty, the inner circle is never located, because no clear solution may be ascertainable from coupling existing knowledge with available data.

Sound decision making requires navigating reliably and efficiently from an initial position of ignorance, through the first two concentric circles, to the inner circle. Reliability and efficiency in this process are crucial. All possibilities relevant to the medical problem must be considered, and from those, all possibilities irrelevant to the individual patient must then be excluded, without unnecessary trial and error.

Another way to visualize these concepts is a grid, with columns for all options and rows for all findings applicable to the problem in question. The grid corresponds to the outer circle depicted above. The positive findings for any individual patient will fill only a small fraction of the cells in the grid, and the pattern formed by those cells (corresponding to the second circle) will differ for almost every patient. When those cells are concentrated in one column, that option may be chosen for that patient (corresponding to the inner circle), but even then different patients in the same column will likely vary—their patterns will mostly overlap but not be identical.

The above process can also be conceived as a calculus of small steps for applying medical knowledge to detailed patient data points. Patients are not rectangles; length and width are insufficient data to describe them. Patients are the shape under a curve. Just as calculus provides a technique for measuring the area under the curve by dividing up that shape infinitesimally, so knowledge coupling is a technique for dividing up a known medical problem into many discrete findings for purposes of matching with detailed patient data.[59]

Once the knowledge coupling process identifies possibilities relevant to the patient, the next step is to prioritize those possibilities for further consideration.

---

59   We will return to this concept of the divisibility of knowledge, which leads to conceiving of knowledge as a network of interconnections among many points. The "Knowledge Net" underlying knowledge coupling software embodies this concept. See the discussions at notes 103, 147, 231-232, and 294 below.

Knowledge coupling software does not establish priorities but groups the possibilities in a way that facilitates judgments about priority. The grouping varies depending on the medical problem involved. For example, the Coupler for diagnosis of hematuria classifies possible diagnoses into the following groups:

- Rapidly Progressing Disorders: May Need Immediate Attention

- Causes for Which Just One Finding Makes Consideration Mandatory

- Other Causes of Hematuria

- Approach for Isolated Hematuria When No Findings Suggest a Diagnosis

Within each one of these groups, the Coupler output lists primary options (e.g., diagnostic possibilities) for which one or more positive findings appear in the patient. For each option, the listing shows the number of positive findings in the patient and the total number of possible findings for that option. That information gives the user an immediate sense of which options seem to best match the patient. For example, the output might show that 5 of 7 findings positive for one option, while only one or two findings are positive for the other options. But the apparent best match should not necessarily be the highest priority option. The highest priority options to consider are rapidly progressing disorders that could cause harm if not treated quickly. The next highest priority group is options for which just one positive finding makes consideration mandatory, regardless of how many positive findings appear for other options. The next group lists other possible options, which can easily be ranked by the positive findings as a proportion of all findings for each option. That numerical ranking, however, is not a sufficient basis for judgment. Also needed is further information about each option, including a description of typical manifestations, known variations from what is typical, epidemiological information about prevalence in various populations, possible tests to order and other information useful for diagnostic assessment. This kind of detail appears when the user clicks on each option in the list.

Sometimes the detailed description for one of the options matches the patient closely, and all other options match poorly. That description might identify a single test to confirm or rule out the option, or, in the absence of such a test, the user may judge whether the option can be accepted as clearly the correct diagnosis. In other cases, several options might be worth considering based on positive findings and the descriptions provided, while in other cases, none of the descriptions match the patient well and no diagnosis seems plausible. In these two situations, the Coupler provides detailed further guidance for each option. In the Hematuria Coupler, for example, under the heading "Approach for Isolated Hematuria When No Findings Suggest a Diagnosis," the following subheadings appear: (1) Isolated hematuria with no plausible diagnosis, (2) Left renal vein hypertension, and (3) Prostatic venous rupture. Under the first subheading the user finds epidemiological information (e.g. cancer and urological disease prevalence among men above and below age 40 with microscopic hematuria) and detailed explanation and references about possible further testing and monitoring. Similar guidance is provided for left renal vein hypertension and prostatic venous rupture.

Another example is the Coupler for management of Type I and II diabetes in adults (including gestational diabetes, disease complications and related conditions). The options are classified into the following groups (only those relevant to an individual patient will be displayed):

- Glucose-Related Crises Requiring Hospitalization

- Related Conditions Requiring Identification and Management

- Monitoring Diabetes Control

- Controlling and Monitoring Diet

- Exercise

- Overview of Drugs for Diabetes

- Oral Drugs That Increase Insulin Secretion by the Pancreas

- Oral Drugs that Decrease Insulin Resistance & Increase Glucose Use

- Oral Drugs that Slow Digestion of Complex Carbohydrates after Meals

- Insulin Therapy

- Before-Meal Insulin Analogs and Inhaled Insulin

- Basal Insulin Analogs

- Insulin Therapy: Preventing and Monitoring For Common Problems

- Foot Care

- Travel Considerations

- Cholesterol and Triglyceride Management

- Blood Pressure Management

- Preventing, Monitoring For, and Managing Associated Conditions

- Pregnancy and Diabetes

- Monitoring for and Managing Complications of Diabetes

- Other Couplers That Might Provide Further Guidance

- Complementary and Alternative Medicine (CAM)

- Emerging Therapies and Therapies of Limited Availability

- Options For Which Only Cautions Are Present*

    * This heading includes guidance options that are unlikely to apply to the particular patient, but for which information about cautions might be useful.

A useful comparison with the combinatorial approach and knowledge coupling software is the concept of simply entering findings into a search engine such as Google.[60] That approach falls far short of knowledge coupling at three levels. First, the search results depend entirely on what terms the user enters in the search engine, that is, on the initial findings the user judges to be significant. That exercise of judgment completely undermines the initial workup. Different combinations of findings initially selected on a patient may point in very different directions. No one can be confident that the right combination of findings will emerge unless the initial workup takes into account, without omission, *all* the findings needed to elicit *all* the options worth considering for the individual patient. Second, Google searches an unfiltered, unstructured body of information—the entire world wide web—completely unlike the distilled and structured body of precisely relevant information in which knowledge coupling "searches" take place. Third, the output of a Google search lacks the structure and precise relevance of the output generated by knowledge coupling software. Accordingly, the cited *BMJ* article on use of Google as a diagnostic aid acknowledged serious limitations in that approach:

We suspect that using Google to search for a diagnosis is likely to be more effective for conditions with unique symptoms and signs that can easily be used as search terms ... Searches are less likely to be successful in complex diseases with non-specific symptoms ... or common diseases with rare presentations ... . The efficiency of the search and the usefulness of the retrieved information also depend on the searchers' knowledge base.

---

60   Tang H, Ng J. Googling for a diagnosis—use of Google as a diagnostic aid: internet based study. BMJ, doi:10.1136/bmj.39003.640567.AE (published 10 November 2006), http://www.bmj.com/cgi/rapidpdf/bmj.39003.640567.AEv1.

Some observers have pointed out that the Internet has created an unprecedented excess of available information. In the past, much of that information would have been forgotten rather than preserved. Now it seems as if "the art of forgetting" must be restored.[61] This new excess of information magnifies a dilemma already inherent in any attempt to apply complex general knowledge to specific problem situations. Sometimes expressed as "connecting the dots," or "finding the needle in a haystack," this dilemma does not require the "art of forgetting." Instead, it requires (1) careful distillation and arrangement of potentially useful knowledge in a specialized repository, and (2) a tool for linking that distilled knowledge with data about specific problem situations, filtering out whatever is extraneous and presenting the rest in maximally usable form for patient care.

PKC Corp. has built a version of the knowledge repository, referred to as the Knowledge Net; PKC's knowledge coupling software is a version of a tool for users to access the repository. Ultimately, the work PKC has done needs to be further developed and become tightly connected to institutions such as the CDC, the FDA and others, institutions that could harvest new knowledge from patient care and then feed that research back into the Knowledge Net. See the diagram in part I. To reiterate, patient care becomes more meaningful for research when the care is documented in problem-oriented records and when inputs to care are informed by knowledge coupling tools (rather than by variable initiative practitioners and their limited ability to keep up to date).

Use of knowledge coupling software does more than locate relevant information; it also changes modes of expression, which in turn changes perception. In traditional practice, a complex patient encounter is typically reduced to a few words or phrases in the record stating the physician's "impression." That impression is bound to be both incomplete and subjective. Moreover, the language chosen to express it may further distort the reality of the patient's condition. It is always the case that language appropriates and alters reality by representing it in terms of the speaker's or writer's perspective, using words and concepts that the audience may understand differently. But with the use of external tools, this process becomes transparent, defined and subject to organized improvement.[62] Rather than have the practitioner compose a selective, minimalist statement of impressions from a limited initial workup (or

---

61 Viktor Mayer-Schönberger, "Useful Void: The Art of Forgetting in the Age of Ubiquitous Computing" (April 2007), http://ksgnotes1.harvard.edu/Research/wpaper.nsf/rwp/RWP07-022/$File/rwp_07_022_mayer-schoenberger.pdf; Seth Lloyd, "You Know Too Much" (4/28/07), http://discovermagazine.com/2007/apr/you-know-too-much.

62 *Knowledge Coupling*, note 2 above, p. 52.

cut and paste some other practitioner's previous text in an electronic record), the combinatorial approach has the patient work with the practitioner to select from pre-defined, careful descriptions of myriad details that might describe the patient's condition. The descriptions from which the patient selects may be pictorial as well as textual. And the patient and practitioner remain free to add their own free-text descriptions on specific points.

It is important to understand that use of Couplers breaks down specialty boundaries. For significant medical problems the outer and middle circles of information encompass multiple specialties. Specialized knowledge inevitably is incomplete and fragmented relative to actual patient needs. As a result, specialist physicians ultimately face the same dilemma as primary care physicians. To reiterate, they cannot know all the tests and observations that might be relevant to complex medical problems. Nor can they know how to interpret and inter-relate all the results. Nor do they have time for the research needed to fill in the gaps in their knowledge. Even when their knowledge is sufficient, physicians are frequently unable to apply their knowledge to detailed data in an organized, reliable manner. For those reasons, failures to collect, comprehend or even keep track of potentially useful data are endemic in medicine. These are not failures of individual physicians. Rather they are failures of a non-system that imposes burdens too great for physicians to bear.

Despite the relief from these burdens that knowledge coupling software provides, some physicians may initially find that its use is disruptive and disturbing. The disruption is in part external, because using Couplers effectively involves changing office procedures and making greater use of non-physician personnel. But the disruption is also internal and thus disturbing, because a change in self-image is involved. The software constantly confronts physicians with options and evidence going beyond what they would take into account if left to their own devices. Physicians soon realize that all their hard-won knowledge is radically incomplete, and often misleading. Entrenched mental habits must change.

It becomes apparent to physicians that their role is not to *learn* medical knowledge but rather to *access and apply* the limited knowledge relevant to each patient's individual needs. Physician co-workers and patients also see the new role. Everyone sees that the new role cannot be performed reliably if the physician exercises clinical judgment about what initial data are worth collecting for each patient. And, as we shall see, everyone finds rewards when the practitioner collects, without omission, all the data made relevant by the outer circle of knowledge, along with any additional data that the practitioner or patient believe are relevant. See part IV.G.4.

G. Answering objections to the combinatorial approach

In light of this basic description of the combinatorial approach and the external tool needed apply it, let us revisit the five objections outlined in part IV.E above.[63] In reading this discussion, keep in mind the three steps of the initial workup (see part IV.B) and the three circles of information (see part IV.F).

1. Feasibility of detailed initial data collection

As we have seen, the tool-driven combinatorial approach requires collecting initial data in far greater detail than is customary. Physicians object that the level of detail involved as prohibitively time-consuming. In many practice settings, physicians are expected to see several patients every hour. That pace leaves no time to collect detailed data, much less time to analyze and review it all with the patient. Even in settings where the pace is slower, physicians may view the combinatorial approach to the initial workup as unacceptably time-consuming.

This objection is not meaningful unless it takes into account the *utility* of the combinatorial approach. The utility of the combinatorial approach is the subject of parts IV.G.2-5 below. If that approach is sufficiently useful in terms of quality and long-run cost-effectiveness, then its time demands should be enforced without regard to the prior habits or expectations or economic demands of providers and third party payers. In this first section, however, we argue that the combinatorial approach is less time consuming and more feasible than it may appear at first glance.

Recall the three steps of the initial workup: choice, collection and analysis of patient data. The practitioner needs to spend *no* time on the first step. The software builders invest immense time on this first step so that the practitioner need not spend any. Moreover, the chosen data points are limited to simple, non-invasive, quick and inexpensive observations and procedures. Non-physician practitioners and patients themselves, guided by knowledge coupling software, can gather those data with great efficiency and reliability.[64] [65] Entering history and symptom data in the software requires the patient to do nothing more than click once (to say "yes") on those findings that the patient recognizes as

---

63   These objections, and the following more detailed statements of them, have not all been articulated by physician users of knowledge coupling software. Rather, the following includes our attempts to anticipate objections and articulate them as well as possible.

64   Bartholomew K. The Perspective of a Practitioner, in Weed LL. et al., *Knowledge Coupling: New Premises and New Tools for Medical Care Education*, New York: Springer-Verlag, 1991, p. 240.

65   Burger, C., "The Use of Problem Knowledge Couplers in a Primary Care Practice", *Healthcare Information Management*, vol. 11, no. 4, Winter 1997, available at www.pkc.com

describing his or her condition (positive findings). The patient clicks twice to say "not sure." Negative findings require no action at all. And most findings are negative for most patients. Most patients thus can rapidly make hundreds of findings simply by paging through computer displays, clicking on the occasional positive or uncertain item. Some findings require the patient to click on a button to review an explanatory graphic or text. That extra step for the patient saves time for the practitioner, because the patient relies on the software for initial help. Moreover, positive and uncertain findings can be annotated with free text when the patient or practitioner wish to elaborate. That extra step also becomes a timesaver, because it elicits and captures significant patient data in context for later use. One practitioner estimates that gathering data in this manner is 5-10 times faster than a verbal discussion covering the same amount of data.[66]

Thus far we have considered choice and collection of data, The efficiency of the combinatorial approach becomes most obvious at step 3 of the initial workup: data analysis, that is, linkage with comprehensive medical knowledge bearing on the significance of the data. With knowledge coupling software, that step occurs instantaneously. Equally important, the software's output organizes all this information for rapid comprehension, while filtering out extraneous information that can safely be ignored. Specifically, the software displays a list of diagnostic or therapeutic options suggested by the initial positive and uncertain findings on the patient (the middle circle of information), while omitting options for which not a single positive finding is made (the outer circle). The options displayed are logically grouped, and clicking on each option displays all of its positive, uncertain and negative findings as evidence for or against that option in that patient, along with additional description, commentary and citations about the option and findings.

This output is generated automatically, without the time-consuming process of drafting or dictating/typing/proofing a narrative summary. The software's output is more complete, organized and precise than a narrative summary and more compatible with coding systems. The output can be printed or exported to electronic medical record systems, and reports can be generated in rich text format for printing or electronic transmission to the patient and other providers. In short, using software tools to couple medical knowledge with patient data generates enormous direct administrative efficiencies. The more important source of efficiency, however, is avoiding unnecessary trial and error.

Using knowledge coupling software for the initial workup resembles use of a map. A map is a highly efficient information tool for navigating in unfamiliar territory. Its efficiency results from its communicating carefully selected

---

66   Personal communication with Harold D. Cross, M.D.

geographic information in a distilled, visual form that is maximally usable at the point of need. Similarly, knowledge coupling software provides a map to the landscape of medical knowledge. Patient-specific data items entered into the software, like coordinates on the X and Y axes of a map, enable the user to find immediately the patient's location in the landscape of medical knowledge.

The practitioner and patient can rapidly compare the patient's condition with more-or-less similar situations described in the software's output The output includes not only the options and data it suggests but also the commentary it provides and the medical literature it cites. Detailed information becomes manageable because it is filtered and organized based on individual relevance to each patient's unique combination of needs.

A careful initial workup is thus much more feasible than it may first appear. As described by a pioneering user of knowledge coupling software, Dr. Ken Bartholomew:

> ... let me dispel the notion that [Couplers] are extremely time-consuming if used properly. Certainly, the first few times using a Coupler will be time consuming, but no more so than reading a textbook chapter on a given problem. ... Because of the timeliness of the data that is built into the couplers, and since they are so pertinent by being problem-oriented [i.e. relevant to presenting problems], I do not need to spend 20 or 30 minutes going through indices of textbooks to find what may or may not be appropriate information.[67]

The whole question of feasibility is thus transformed. Once external tools are employed, nothing less than detailed data collection seems feasible for individualized problem solving.

Moreover, knowledge coupling software makes it feasible to increase reliance on inexpensive non-physician practitioners. As described by one user of knowledge coupling software, Dr. Charles Burger:

> We have trained medical assistants to a high level of skill in information gathering and physical examination. They serve as the main information gatherers, entering historical and physical examination findings into the coupler. Since couplers define the universe of what needs to be done for each problem, the medical assistants become extremely skillful in these basic but important tasks. This use of medical assistants allows the physician or nurse practitioner to spend most of his or her time clarifying

---

67   Bartholomew K. The Perspective of a Practitioner, in Weed LL et al, *Knowledge Coupling: New Premises and New Tools for Medical Care Education*, New York: Springer-Verlag, 1991, p. 240.

and annotating the history, checking certain physical findings, and, most important, reviewing the results of the coupler session with the patient to make decisions regarding possible diagnoses or management options.[68]

Similarly, as described by Dr. Bartholomew:

In my clinic we have experimented with nurses ... doing the "pre-workup." This is the bulk of the time-consuming process. When I enter the examining room, I have a coupler [output] that is largely done. With a good nurse, a large portion of the common physical findings can be entered in the computer and a note left if something is in question. The physician then rechecks any physical findings that are positive or questionable. This is, in fact, extremely time saving and allows you to ... "become a consultant in your own practice."

Couplers are invaluable not only for clinical practitioners but also for receptionists who receive calls from patients seeking care for new medical problems. Handling these calls is a triage function requiring significant medical expertise. In order to provide that expertise to his office staff, Dr. Charles Burger has spent more than 20 years developing, using and refining customized knowledge coupling software (a "triage Coupler"). Receptionists (their title is patient service representative) are trained to use this Coupler. They rely on it to determine:

1) whether the patient needs to be seen in the office, and if so, how soon; 2) how much time should be allowed for the visit; and 3) whether any testing should be done before the visit. In many cases, patient service representatives can provide advice and treatment to be followed at home, saving the patient an office visit. Patients with life-threatening symptoms may be told to go directly to an Emergency Department.

The triage Coupler has been further developed to provide guidance on medication refills and routine problems such as uncomplicated urinary tract infections in women, and treatment for documented strep infections. Like other Couplers, the triage Coupler is periodically reviewed and updated, incorporating user feedback and new findings from the medical literature. Dr. Burger and his colleagues have found that the triage Coupler is beneficial to the morale of both

---

68   Burger, Charles S., "The Use of Problem Knowledge Couplers in a Primary Care Practice," note 2 above, p. 19. The physician who authored this 1997 article has described his current practice in the Spring 2010 issue of *The Permanente Journal*, 14:1;47-50, at http://xnet.kp.org/permanentejournal/spr10/ProblemKnowledgeCouplers.pdf.

the clinical practitioners (whose workload is better managed) and the patient service representatives (who are empowered with expertise to help patients).

Moreover, practitioners who organize their practices to take advantage of knowledge coupling software for triage, screening, diagnosis and treatment/management may find significant economic benefits.[69] And the rewards are more than economic. Use of knowledge coupling software lessens physician burdens and makes practice more interesting and satisfying. As described by Dr. Bartholomew:

> The physician in this setting enters the equation at a higher level of expertise, and, instead of spending the whole day gathering mundane data, spends much more time reviewing the complexities of the cases that need that extra caution to the patient's benefit. Furthermore, I must admit that the practice of medicine in this setting is simply more fun. It is more fun because it is more intellectually rewarding, and this is itself an excellent reason to be using couplers. By having this extra time to spend on more complex cases, the physician can then begin to use the couplers to function at a higher intellectual level than a busy practice usually affords. ...
>
> ... The couplers are full of information; I have never failed to learn something new each time I have used one. ... Using couplers begins to become a reinforcing loop—because they are fun to use, you use them more. The more you realize that valuable information, beyond your own personal store of knowledge, is being brought to bear on each of the patient's problems, the more secure you feel, the more patient gratification you generate, and the more gratification you have from your own practice.[70]

The foregoing addresses the feasibility and benefits of the combinatorial approach from the physician's perspective. But in the long run that is the wrong perspective. Medicine's division of labor needs to shift away from the physician and towards external information tools, non-physician practitioners, and patients themselves. That conclusion becomes increasingly obvious as we further address physician objections to the combinatorial approach.

---

69   Documentation of the economic benefits is provided in Burger, C. "A Coupler Centered Practice: Business Case Analysis for Couplers," available at http://www.pkc.com/papers/ccp3.pdf. The above description of the triage Coupler is from the *Permanante Journal* article cited in the preceding note and personal communications with Dr. Burger. As this article describes, patients frequently complete the medical history portion of Couplers from their homes, using a Web portal to access the Couplers.

70   Bartholomew, note 67 above, p. 240.

2. Utility of detailed initial data

Physicians tend to question whether detailed data collection is truly productive at the outset of care. The only advantage of detailed initial data, it seems, is identifying as many diagnostic or therapeutic options as possible. Most of those possibilities will turn out to be inapplicable to any individual patient (i.e. located in the outer circle of information, as described in part IV.F). Physicians believe that their expertise enables them to leapfrog over the outer circle. They can rapidly identify the options of probable relevance to the individual patient. Those are the options worth investigating (the middle circle), and only limited data are needed to identify them, physicians believe. The important question, on this view, is whether objective evidence of probability, rather than subjective, variable physician judgments, should be the basis for identifying the options worth investigating. Whatever the answer to that question may be, expert physicians collect initial data selectively rather than exhaustively. If and when it becomes necessary to investigate improbable options (rare diagnoses, non-standard treatments), then more detailed data collection may be needed and specialists may be consulted. An iterative process of successive elimination thus occurs. On this view, collecting detailed initial data at the outset of care defeats a primary purpose of expert functioning in the initial workup—to avoid unnecessary data collection.[71]

This entire point of view rests on a mistaken premise—that detailed initial data collection is not needed to identify the options worth investigating. The reality, however, is the opposite. The only reliable way to determine the options worth investigating *for an individual patient* is first to collect patient-specific data in great detail.

Much of the detailed initial data will indeed turn out to be irrelevant. But the relevant and irrelevant data cannot be distinguished in advance. They vary for each patient with the same presenting problem. Detailed data must therefore be gathered at the outset. In no other way is it possible to identify all options of potential relevance, and narrow them down to options of actual relevance, for an individual patient. These threshold inquiries are compromised when detailed data collection and analysis are deferred.

"The matter of time is essential in all estimates of the value of information," Norbert Wiener once observed.[72] In medicine, the value of detailed information

---

71   This section draws on "The Database," in *Knowledge Coupling*, and on *The Philosophy, Use and Interpretation of Knowledge Couplers*, note 2 above, co-authored and authored, respectively, by Chris Weed.

72   N. Wiener. *The Human Use of Human Beings.* Boston: Houghton Mifflin, 1950, 1954; New York: Avon Books, 1967, p. 168.

is greater at the outset of care than the value of the *same* information gathered piecemeal, over time. That reality explains the traditional precept (honored more in the breach than the observance) that a detailed patient history "is still the most essential part of clinical decision making. ... Extra time spent gathering data almost always saves much more time in the long run."[73]

This observation from 20 years ago is now true more than ever, because growing medical knowledge increases the utility of data available from a well-designed patient history (as well as physical examination and basic laboratory tests). As Dr. Ami Schattner has written: "Diagnostic difficulties can often be resolved by simple means. ... close attention to the safest, least expensive, and most informative test of all—the history—can help resolve diagnostic and therapeutic dilemmas weeks and sometimes months before they might otherwise be resolved."[74] Moreover, the patient history, physical exam and basic laboratory tests may be needed to use advanced diagnostic tests productively, in both formulating inquiries and interpreting results. For example, Jerome Groopman points out that the settings for multidetector CT scans (which enable rapid scans of large volumes of tissue) can be adjusted to take into account not just the specific question posed by the referring physician but also the patient's history.[75]

One would hope that economic pressures would induce more effective patient histories and more selective use of costly diagnostic technologies. Dr. Denis Cortese of the Mayo Clinic argues that more selective testing is promoted by sharing of expertise: "' When doctors put their heads together in a room, when they share expertise, you get more thinking and less testing.'"[76] Sharing expertise is what knowledge coupling software accomplishes. The sharing occurs automatically from use of the tools, and the expertise built into the tools goes far beyond the expertise and thinking of physicians who get together in a room.

Nothing of this kind has occurred in the marketplace. As Dr. Schattner observes: "physicians have become 'fascinated', 'preoccupied' and 'obsessed' with their new instruments," which "are vigorously promoted by the large companies that supply them." This state of affairs is destructive at many levels:

With the increasing availability of powerful diagnostic instruments, physicians have become distanced from both their patients and the basic clinical data. Today, tests and procedures are considered infallible

73   Mold, JW, Stein JF. The cascade effect in the clinical care of patients. *New England Journal of Medicine*, 1986. 314:512-14 (p. 513).

74   Schattner A. "Simple Is Beautiful: The Neglected Power of Simple Tests." Arch Intern Med 164: 2198-2200 at 2199 (Nov. 8, 2004).

75   Groopman J., *How Doctors Think*, note 11 above, pp. 193-94.

76   Quoted in Gawande, A. The Cost Conundrum. *The New Yorker*, June 1, 2009.

and ordered in increasing numbers—often almost blindly, repeatedly and sometimes even without examining the patient. Thus, many are redundant, inconclusive or misleading, in addition to being unnecessarily expensive. Uncertainty, false positive findings and fear of lawsuits often beget more tests or procedures and may trigger dangerous cascades. This testing-dominated approach undermines the value of clinical skills, which tend to become underestimated, underused and finally lost.[77]

A primary reason for neglect of basic clinical observations and tests is their multiplicity. That makes it difficult to know or recall what tests are available for any given problem or which tests should be used when. Equally difficult is comprehending all the data generated. Accordingly, Dr. Schattner argues, fully exploiting information from the patient history "mandates a closely linked and thoughtful use of large, preferably electronic, databases." But Dr. Schattner does not address the core issues of how and when external databases are to be used. In traditional medical practice, the physician's unaided mind largely determines the content of the initial history during the patient encounter; afterwards the physician may go to medical libraries and electronic databases for external guidance, if time permits. This sequence is backwards. External software tools enable guidance to be organized *before* and used *during* the three steps of the initial workup—choice, collection and analysis of patient data. *Then* the practitioner and patient may supplement the software's output with additional observations suggested by their personal knowledge, experience and judgment—that of the practitioner who may have seen many other similar patients, and that of the patient whose intimate personal knowledge and experience of her own condition may reveal crucial variations from what is expected.

The preceding discussion is framed in terms of diagnostic decision making, but a similar analysis applies to treatment decision making, especially management of chronic disease. Many problems require considering a multiplicity of treatment options, including expensive technologies, a variety of medications, other interventions and changes in patient behaviors. Evaluating the options for each individual patient requires detailed data collection and analysis. Without

---

77   Schattner, A. "Clinical paradigms revisited," *Medical Journal of Australia*, 2006; 185 (5): 273-275, available at http://www.mja.com.au/public/issues/185_05_040906/sch10143_fm.html. See also Dr. Schattner's response to letters to the editor, criticizing "imaging without forethought." *Ibid*, 2006; 185 (11/12): 671-672 [Letters], available at http://www.mja.com.au/public/issues/185_11_041206/arn11029_letters_fm-2.html. It is remarkable that these issues are still the subject of debate. By now it should be obvious that practitioners need information tools to use clinical imaging tools effectively as much as they need the imaging tools to reveal internal organs. In both contexts, ignoring modern technology is unacceptable.

the necessary standards and tools, patient needs are easily sacrificed to the short-term economic interests of other parties.

This notion that routinely collecting detailed data is useful may seem to contradict research in the psychology of decision making. Summarizing this research, Malcolm Gladwell states that in some situations "you need to know very little to find the underlying signature of a complex phenomenon." In such cases, Gladwell concludes, collecting and considering detailed data bury the few data points that matter in a mass of extraneous information.[78] This point is valid as far as it goes, but it overlooks two crucial elements. First, when many possibilities must be considered and each one has a different signature (e.g., multiple diagnostic possibilities, each with its own cluster of findings), then detailed data must be collected in order to consider all the possibilities. Second, finding the few data points that matter buried within detailed information is readily accomplished with software tools. Breaking our dependence on the unaided mind solves the needle-in-a-haystack problem.

The Addison's disease case discussed in Part II.A powerfully illustrates these points. Recall that the physicians began by considering only a limited range of diagnostic options, based on probabilities: "the clinician usually begins a diagnostic investigation by considering (and excluding) the *most common* diagnoses. As those most common diagnoses become less likely, many *less common* diagnoses are considered" (emphasis added).[79] Consistent with this accepted practice, an evidence-based ranking of diagnostic possibilities for fatigue would assign a low rank to Addison's disease, because that condition is rare, both in the general population and in the population of patients with severe fatigue.

But those broad populations were not relevant for this particular patient. Instead, relevant to her was the limited group of individuals with combinations of findings similar to hers (even if each finding is non-specific). The initial findings on her included fatigue, shortness of breath, hypotension, weight loss and numerous, deeply pigmented moles—each of which are documented manifestations of Addison's disease. Soon after the initial encounter, additional known signs and symptoms of Addison's disease appeared. In the limited group of patients with such a combination of findings, Addison's disease should be ranked high as a probable diagnosis. But in this case it was not even considered as a possibility until the patient was near death.

In beginning with the most common possibilities, physicians commit a basic conceptual error. Indeed, this approach is backwards. What is common or rare

---

78   Gladwell, M. *Blink* (New York: Little Brown and Co., 2005), pp. 136-45.
79   Keljo D, Squires R. note 3 above (p. 48).

in the general population should be the last information to consider, not the first. The first information to consider *for an individual patient* should be all the possible diagnoses suggested by the patient's particular combination of findings, regardless of the probability of those diagnoses occurring in larger populations. Addison's disease would have immediately emerged as a highly probable diagnosis if the non-specific findings on this girl were *combined*. The underlying principle is clear: findings that are non-specific when viewed in isolation often become highly specific when viewed in combination. A corollary principle is that judgments of probability are highly misleading as applied to individual patients. Those judgments are derived from large population studies where the few variables examined become isolated from the detailed patient data needed for combinatorial analysis.

These principles give the combinatorial approach enormous power. But that power depends on gathering data in sufficient detail and then reliably matching it with medical knowledge. The reliability of both tasks depends on using software tools rather than the unaided mind to guide initial data collection and analysis.

Data collection guided by software tools is highly standardized. Why mandate that departure from accepted practice?

3. Utility of standardized initial data

Physicians tend to object that the combinatorial approach does not allow for case-by-case discretionary judgments in selecting initial data. This view rejects a central element of the combinatorial approach—that *standardized* initial data must be determined in advance for a given presenting problem. In other words, for every patient who has that problem, the practitioner must habitually collect all data specified in advance, without any omissions based on the practitioner's clinical judgment. To some physicians, this standardization is mere "cookbook medicine."

This view is backwards. In reality, cookbook medicine results from our human propensity to process only information that supports our preconceptions. Each physician has a personal set of preconceptions. The only systemic protection from these variable personal cookbooks is to standardize initial data collection and analysis.

Paradoxically, *standardized* data collection is essential to capturing the *uniqueness* of individual patients. Their medical individuality emerges when data are consistently collected from a predefined universe with sufficient detail to show individual variations. In contrast, when physicians have discretion to shorten a standardized initial workup, key individual variations may be lost.

Consider, for example, the problem of diabetes management. An initial workup should cover some 330 findings. Each patient's set of positive findings will differ. And those variations among diabetic patients may be crucial to their care, because every finding is carefully selected in advance for its direct relevance to diabetes management. If physicians substitute their own judgments for the predefined initial workup, some of those judgments will result in omissions. And some of those omissions will reflect physician idiosyncrasies (time constraints, specialty, unsupported hypotheses) rather than accurate judgments of which findings can safely be ignored. In short, allowing judgmental *omissions* from a predefined initial workup reintroduces the very idiosyncrasies that patients need protection against. (Judgmental *additions* to the initial workup are a quite different matter, as discussed below.)

Some experienced physicians may be confident that they can judge when it is safe to abbreviate an initial workup. Their talent and experience, they believe, often enable them to recognize the correct diagnosis or treatment without performing a complete workup. But those physicians also view their judgments as superior to those of other physicians with less talent or experience, and certainly superior to the judgments of non-physicians. Permitting those *other* practitioners to omit portions of the initial workup at their discretion will therefore, superior physicians must concede, leave patients at risk. Moreover, even the most self-confident physicians must also concede that their superior judgments will not always be accepted on faith by patients or others. Indeed, patients or colleagues or payers or regulators might prefer to rely on initial workups conducted by non-physician practitioners, who would not presume to cut corners during the initial workup based on their personal knowledge or judgment.

In short, everyone involved needs some objective standard for identifying trustworthy judgments. The combinatorial approach provides the necessary objective standard—that is, detailed patient data selected in advance based on review of the medical literature. Patients or others who are unwilling to accept physician judgments on faith can simply demand completion of the predefined initial workup, even if the physician views it as unnecessary overkill. A self-confident physician should welcome that demand, because a complete initial workup presumably will vindicate his superior judgment—that is, the physician will have already considered anything significant the complete initial workup reveals.

Actual experience with the combinatorial approach reveals that the self-confidence of even the best physicians is often misplaced. The human mind, no matter how gifted and well-schooled, simply cannot be trusted with the intricate information processing that individualized decision making entails. When the medical literature shows that 300+ initial findings are needed to manage diabetes, for example, the physician's case-by-case judgments of when to dispense with some of those findings are bound to be fallible. Every patient's combination of findings will vary. Any individual variation may turn out to be significant. And this differentiation increases with chronic conditions, as each patient's evolving disease interacts with his or her unique physiology, psyche and circumstances over time. Any one physician's personal experience with this patient variation is limited. Knowledge coupling software, however, can take into account the accumulated experience of thousands of practitioners and millions of patients.

Moreover, two other factors mandate rigorous enforcement of a combinatorial minimum standard. First, however justifiable some omissions from the initial workup might seem, they create an unexplained gap in the patient's record of care. Practitioners other than the initial examiner cannot distinguish between findings that were checked and found to be negative and findings that were simply omitted and never checked. The resulting uncertainty invites either wasteful duplication or uninformed follow-up.

Second, omissions contaminate the patient's record of care as a source of data for discovering new knowledge. The recorded care of many thousands of patients should provide reliable data from which patterns can be identified, as we shall discuss further in Parts VI and VII.

These points are a reminder that medicine needs something like standards of accounting in the business world. In a business, every deposit and every payment of funds must be recorded. No one would attempt to judge when it is unnecessary to do so, because everyone understands that recording each deposit and payment is essential to maintaining controls over financial operations. Similarly, in medicine, checking every positive finding of a predefined data set is necessary to maintain reliable systems for decision making and feedback. A combinatorial approach to the initial workup makes this point obvious, because it means that each item of data has been carefully chosen in advance for its potential utility.

Here users may reasonably object that they need some flexibility in the timing of data collection for some items (primarily lab tests). It may not always be practical to immediately obtain each and every test result that the knowledge coupling software identifies as needed for the initial workup. The software accommodates this need by designating certain items as data to be collected "if available." When necessary, the user can defer collection of these items in the hope that other data will be enough to arrive at a solution. The key point to recognize is that the software should make this exercise of judgment by the user transparent. The missing data items are recorded as uncertain findings, not as negative findings. Anyone reviewing the Coupler output is thus alerted to the possible need to obtain the missing data. Subsequent researchers can study records of these cases with others where the data are collected to assess its utility.

4. Effect on the doctor-patient relationship

Whatever utility the combinatorial approach to the initial workup may have, physicians still object that it harms their relationship with patients. The combinatorial approach means that the patient interacts initially not with the physician but with a computer and with non-physician personnel who conduct the physical examination. This division of labor is unacceptable to some physicians and patients. They contrast an idealized scenario where the physician sympathetically inquires about the patient's history, personally performs the physical exam, observes the patient's demeanor and immediately orders tests and procedures he judges to be relevant. Through this interaction, it is believed, the physician develops personal rapport, observes firsthand the patient's physical and emotional condition, and establishes his immediate command of the situation.

Physicians are right that their personal relationships with patients are critical. At its best, the human interaction between practitioner and patient is itself therapeutic. But physicians' idealized image of their relationship with patients is hardly consistent with how the initial workup is usually conducted. Time constraints often prevent a careful or sympathetic discussion of the patient's condition, cultural barriers may hinder communication, graduate medical education fosters behaviors and attitudes that interfere with communication, and not all physicians have good communication skills to begin with. In short, the personal relationship between the physician and patient is not necessarily a positive element. Moreover, that personal relationship provides no comfort to patients if not backed by professional expertise the patient can trust.

Patients need to be able to trust the physician to gather and correctly take into account the right information. An objective basis for trust arises when physicians employ a combinatorial approach to the initial workup implemented with software tools. In contrast, a judgmental approach to the initial workup hardly inspires patient trust. "The average patient visiting a doctor in the United States gets 22 seconds for his initial statement, then the doctor takes the lead,"[80]

---

80   Langevitz W, Denz M, Keller A, et al. "Spontaneous talking time at start of consultation in outpatient clinic: cohort study." *BMJ* 2002. 325:682-693.

according to one study. Other observers conclude that the physicians are deficient in bringing out patients' own concerns.[81] This state of affairs fosters cynicism among patients. As expressed in the headline of a New York *Times* article on the subject: "Tell the Doctor All Your Problems, But Keep It to Less Than a Minute." The hurried, judgmental approach remains accepted practice even though research has "linked poor communication to misdiagnoses, the ordering of unnecessary tests, and the failure of patients to follow treatment plans."[82]

Critics of current practice advocate improved interviewing techniques by physicians.[83] Yet, no improvements in interviewing will ever bring initial workups to an acceptable level of quality. So long as physician judgment determines the content of the workup, the inevitable outcome is enormous variation from one physician to another. Drs. John Bjorn and Harold Cross documented this phenomenon more than 35 years ago[84] when they recruited one of their patients to take her case to a number of physicians in their community. This patient found that each physician elicited different information and drew different conclusions, even though they were examining the same symptoms in the same person.

Since then, innumerable studies have further documented that variation among providers is the norm in numerous medical contexts (most of these studies do not examine the context of the initial workup, the importance of which is not generally recognized). These studies, however, typically do not compare responses of different providers to a single patient but rather compare provider responses to a single disease condition. Variation is conceived as departure from "evidence-based" guidelines for a particular disease condition. This concept does not account for the possibility that some variations by physicians justifiably reflect the varying needs of individual patients labeled with the "same" disease. In contrast, the Bjorn and Cross study, by comparing responses of multiple physicians to a single patient, clearly shows that variation reflects provider idiosyncrasies. This conclusion comes as no surprise to patients.

Patients and doctors are adrift. For them, the system fails even to define the optimal initial workup, much less disseminate and enforce it. This state of affairs is what harms the doctor-patient relationship. Patients see that physicians'

---

81   *Ibid.*; Marvel MK, Epstein RM, Flowers K, Beckman HB. Soliciting the patient's agenda: have we improved? *JAMA* 1999. 281:283-287.

82   M. Levine, "Tell the Doctor All Your Problems, but Keep It to Less Than a Minute." New York Times, June 1, 2004.

83   *Ibid.*; Marvel MK, Epstein RM, Flowers K, Beckman HB. Soliciting the patient's agenda: have we improved? *JAMA* 1999. 281:283-287.

84   Bjorn J, Cross H. *The Problem-Oriented Private Practice of Medicine.* 1970. Chicago: Modern Healthcare Press, pp. 24-28.

initial workups are variable, ad hoc and incomplete. The patient is too often left wondering whether the physician considered all the relevant diagnostic or treatment possibilities, gathered the right data, correctly interpreted the data obtained, and carefully recorded what was done. Physicians themselves may have the same doubts about their own work, and that of their colleagues (which is one reason why patients find themselves repeatedly asked for the same data). The result is that patients shuttle from one costly specialist to another, because no one involved can tell whether the uncertainty they face reflects gaps in personal knowledge (which the next specialist might know enough to remedy), or whether that uncertainty reflects gaps in current medical science (which makes the next specialist consultation an exercise in futility).

This disorder undermines the therapeutic benefit inherent in caregiving itself. Medical attention satisfies a basic human need for sympathy and relief. But if patients perceive disorder and lack of care in what is done to them, that perception alone may destroy the therapeutic benefit that caregiving itself potentially confers.

Unlike a judgmental approach to the initial workup, an orderly, combinatorial approach lays a secure foundation for a system of trust. Both practitioners and patients feel protected against the limits and idiosyncrasies of the unaided mind. Uncertainty is reduced, and open communication is enhanced. The combinatorial approach brings both greater effectiveness and greater honesty to the practitioner's work. As Dr. Richard Rockefeller has written of his experiences in patient care using knowledge coupling software: "our sense of worth and competence is better served by improved outcomes in the realm of the possible than by compensatory fantasies of omniscience."[85] Similarly, Dr. Jerome Groopman (not a user of knowledge coupling software) has written:

> Does acknowledging uncertainty undermine a patient's sense of hope and confidence in his physician and the proposed therapy? Paradoxically, taking uncertainty into account can enhance a physician's therapeutic effectiveness, because it demonstrates his honesty, his willingness to be the more engaged with his patients, his commitment to the reality of the situation rather than resorting to evasion, half-truth and even lies. And it makes it easier for the doctor to change course if the first strategy fails, to keep trying. Uncertainty sometimes is essential for success.[86]

But without knowledge coupling software, it is difficult to distinguish between genuine uncertainty and mere personal unawareness of applicable knowledge.

85 *Knowledge Coupling*, note 2 above, p. ix.
86 Groopman J., note 11 above, p. 155.

A sociologist has done a survey of patient attitudes towards use of PKC knowledge coupling software in a primary care practice.[87] He found that a majority viewed their experience favorably, a significant minority were neutral and a significant minority viewed their experience unfavorably. Elements of the experience that were viewed favorably included thoroughness and depth of data collection, inclusion of personal lifestyle details bearing on diagnostic and treatment decisions, lessened reliance on the doctor's personal knowledge, objective presentation of decision options and evidence, and printouts of the detailed knowledge coupling results (which facilitate recall, understanding, follow-up, and discussion with family members and other providers). Unfavorable reactions appeared to reflect antipathy to computers and a preference for the familiar, personal questioning by an authoritative physician. The sociologist who conducted the survey wrote that some patients view the computer as "fostering an 'impersonal' environment" even though the software elicited detailed findings about the patient's condition and personal circumstances. Also problematic for a few patients is the fact that use of computers protects against the mind's fallibility: "Whereas most respondents applaud this, a few, ironically, seemed disheartened by the tacit admission of the mind's limitations, [which] seemed to diminish their confidence in the care and advice being delivered."[88] A contrasting view was expressed by one of the survey respondents, who commented:

> I have had a couple of problems that a series of doctors failed miserably to diagnose. None of them ever picked up a book while I was in the office nor hinted that they consulted any reference. Perhaps their performance wouldn't have been so pitiful if they had used references. Computers can be a quick way to find and check information.[89]

Dr. Ken Bartholomew, who pioneered use of PKC knowledge coupling software to implement the combinatorial approach, described the trust engendered among his patients:

> Not only do patients see the thoroughness involved in the use of couplers, but they sense that we care enough to give them the kind of thoroughness that they feel entitled to. With the coupler's systematic review of details in the patient's life that could be relevant to the current problem, the patient feels that his or her individual situation has been thoroughly

---

87   Weaver R. "Informatics Tools and Medical Communication: Patient Perspectives of "Knowledge Coupling" in Primary Care," *Health Communication*, 15(1), 59–78 (2003).

88   *Ibid.*, p. 75.

89   *Ibid.* p. 73.

examined and all possible conclusions have been taken into account. In management couplers, they further see the many different combinations of therapy and understand that the care of a complex, long term problem requires a detailed understanding of the patient's unique situation, followed by a careful monitoring of the options chosen. Even when a diagnosis is still in question, they have, in my experience, been completely satisfied with the outcome of the encounter. In addition, by receiving a printout of the findings and possible causes, they feel empowered to review the situation at home and to watch for signs and symptoms that may aid the diagnostic process in the days or weeks to come. The use of couplers teaches them that there is a time course to disease and that not all signs and symptoms necessarily occur "by the book" or simultaneously. By thus empowering our patients with information, as opposed to leaving them in a void, we reinforce their collaborative role as part of a team working toward an understood goal. ... it is only when this occurs that the optimum physician/patient relationship is built.[90]

Another physician user of knowledge coupling software, Dr. Richard Rockefeller, further described the importance to patients of detailed data collection about their personal situations and experiences:

In the prevailing medical paradigm, orientated as it is toward general knowledge, patients feel appreciated and well cared for to the extent that their problems are generic, that is, match population-based classifications of pathology. When the dimensions of their suffering and needs extravasate beyond these borders, as commonly happens, patients discover their idiosyncrasies to be sources of frustration and anger. They often find themselves alienated not only from a system which fails to meet their needs but also from themselves, to the extent they identify with the systems implicit devaluation of their uniqueness. [In contrast, the combinatorial] approach ... takes the set of attributes, historical circumstances and preferences which differentiate one individual from the next as central to, rather than as a troublesome distraction from, the important work of the therapeutic encounter. Patients' satisfaction is enhanced as their aptitudes and contributions—self-knowledge, willingness and ability to gather data pertaining to the problem, among others—are appropriately valued. Finally, as a reward for relinquishing the comfortable (but also dangerous, increasingly untenable and ultimately unfulfilling) illusion of

90   *Knowledge Coupling*, note 2 above, pp. 238-39.

being wholly provided for by an omnipotent parent, patients are afforded the human rewards of collegiality, including equal stature in the patient/doctor relationship and control over decisions affecting their health.[91]

Writing in 1991, long before current discussion of "consumer-driven care," "information therapy" and the like, Dr. Bartholomew and Dr. Rockefeller presciently described an ideal that the marketplace is beginning to recognize. But the recognition is incomplete, and the necessary tools and standards of care are yet to be accepted.

5. Information processing, clinical judgment and the two stages of decision making

Our only remaining hope and salvation is to begin the whole labour of the mind again; not leaving it to itself, but directing it perpetually from the very first, and attaining our end as it were by mechanical aid.

— Francis Bacon[92]

We have seen that clinical judgment is unreliable in both selection and analysis of initial patient data, and we have examined *selection* of initial data at some length. Here we further examine *analysis* of patient data.

a. Analysis as information processing

By "analysis" of patient data we mean a simple process of association between data items and corresponding medical knowledge—for example, the association between a cluster of patient findings and a diagnosis explaining those findings, or the association between possible treatments for the diagnosis and findings bearing on suitability of each treatment for that patient. Conceived in this way, data analysis involves raw information processing—establishing linkages between patient findings and a database of medical knowledge. That function is readily carried out with software tools used by all practitioners and patients themselves. This simple concept of analysis is to be distinguished from more complex processes involving logic and inference. In turn, both simple and complex analytical processes of decision making may be distinguished from instinctive, intuitive processes.

Physicians object that a simple process of association is crude and incomplete. The perceived analytical sophistication involved in understanding patho-

---

91   *Ibid.*, p. ix.

92   Bacon F. *Novum Organon* (1620), Preface to Second Part, available at   http://history.hanover.edu/texts/Bacon/novpref.htm.

physiology is lacking. Moreover, even if software tools with that sophistication were designed, those tools could never capture the subtleties of personal interactions with patients and the resulting instinctive element of clinical judgment.

The reality, however, is that giving free rein to clinical judgment degrades analysis of initial data. Inevitably, physicians jump to conclusions based on skimpy data and limited personal knowledge. As Dr. Jerome Groopman has written of diagnostic analysis, for example, "research shows that most doctors quickly come up with two or three possible diagnoses within minutes of meeting a patient ... All develop their hypotheses from a very incomplete body of information."[93] Their analyses are similarly incomplete in the treatment context, where physicians often fail to consider much of the information needed for identifying and choosing among available treatment options.

The exercise of judgment naturally leads physicians to shortcut crucial threshold processes and plunge into follow-up processes prematurely (recall the distinction between threshold and follow-up processes from part IV.A). Without a secure foundation, those follow-up processes are piecemeal, disorderly, risky and full of waste. Acting in a hit-or-miss fashion, physicians order tests and treatments as soon as possible. If they do not hit on a solution, more tests and treatments are tried. They readily take credit if the patient's condition improves, without acknowledging that the body's internal mechanisms for healing and self-repair might account for the improvement. The escalating volume of data to ponder often becomes too large and disorganized to take it all into account, while the volume of medical knowledge relevant to interpreting all that data becomes too large to recall or comprehend. Coordination, follow-through and feedback frequently fall apart. Risk of mishap lurks every step of the way.

This quagmire traps both primary care physicians and the specialists they consult. A vivid illustration is the Addison's disease case discussed in part II.A. In that case, what was needed was not sophisticated clinical reasoning but simply pattern recognition—the association between the initial findings and the correct diagnosis. Software tools would have been superior to expert judgment for that limited task.

Autonomous clinical judgment is not capable of performing that task reliably, no matter how well physicians are educated. The mind's limited capacity for information processing weakens clinical judgment. To cope with complexity, the mind's normal modes of operation include various simplifying approaches (heuristics) that limit the information taken into account, as decades of research in cognitive psychology have demonstrated. In the last decade, thanks to the patient safety movement, medicine has woken up to the implications of this

93 Groopman J. *How Doctors Think*, note 11 above, p. 35. Recall our earlier discussion at notes 80-83 about doctors' hurried approach to communicating with their patients.

research for explaining why execution of medical decisions so often goes awry. More recently, implications for medical decision making itself have become the focus of attention.[94]

But the weaknesses of clinical judgment go beyond the mental heuristics on which the mind relies to cope with complexity. The problem is also that judgment is idiosyncratic and personal. Except in the simplest matters, no two people take into account the same information in the same way. Idiosyncratic variations among physicians arise from varying individual abilities, varying medical backgrounds (training, experience, specialty orientation), other influences (emotional, cultural and financial), and other contingencies (the time available at the patient encounter, the stage of the patient's condition at that point, the patient's recall of needed information, the interpersonal dynamics between patient and practitioner, the sequence in which different specialists happen to be consulted).

Most of us try to use our judgment to recognize and overcome internal cognitive weaknesses and external influences. But our capacity to do so is just as limited as our capacity to process detailed information. The mental heuristics identified by cognitive psychologists "appear to be integral components of human information processing. As with visual illusions, awareness does not prevent us from being susceptible to their effects ..."[95] Much the same can be said of other influences (financial interests, emotional needs, cultural preconceptions) that further distort judgment. Inevitably, reliance on judgment compromises analysis of initial data.

b. The two stages of decision making and the proper role of judgment

What, then, is the role of judgment, if any, under the combinatorial approach? Recall that decision making can be conceived in two distinct stages: (1) building an informational foundation designed to identify options for decision with the pros and cons of each option, and (2) choosing among the options (see Part III.A at note 38). The first stage requires processing information— retrieval, linkage and sorting of general knowledge and patient-specific data in order to recognize medically significant patterns and relationships. The second stage involves applying judgment to choose among the options in light of the evidence.

---

94   Well before the patient safety movement made the issue prominent, however, the implications of cognitive psychology for medical decision making were discussed in the literature. See the citations and discussion in Weed LL., Physicians of the Future, note 51 above; Weed LL. *Knowledge Coupling*, note 2 above, pp. 8, 37-42, 212, 226-27.

95   A Elstein. Heuristics and Biases: Selected Errors in Clinical Reasoning. *Acad. Med.* 74:791-793 (1999), p. 793.

Judgment at this second stage involves logical analysis, intuition and personal values.

The role of human judgment should be to *supplement* external tools in the first stage of decision making and to *govern* the second stage. In the first stage, the predefined initial workup may be supplemented with additional information judged by the patient or practitioner to be relevant. But judgment should not be permitted to cut short the initial workup. The first stage must be completed, so that, in the second stage, judgment is informed and its basis is transparent. In the second stage, it is the patient's judgment, not the physician's, that should be decisive.

If patient data are carefully chosen in advance, collected without omission and reliably coupled with medical knowledge at the initial workup, then the need for judgment in some cases is almost eliminated. That happens when the first stage reveals a clear solution to the patient's problem. A clear solution is one that anyone's judgment would accept. The Addison's disease case study discussed above provides an example. There, assembling the right information would have revealed a clearly correct diagnosis and treatment at the outset of care, with minimal judgment required. In such cases, the locus of decision making authority should not matter, because the right decision almost makes itself once the right information is assembled.

Significant judgment is needed only if uncertainty remains and opinions vary after rigorous information gathering and processing at the initial workup are completed. At that point, the patient and practitioner are usually faced with a range of possible diagnostic or treatment options to investigate further and choose among. Uncertainty means that no one option stands out as superior to all the others. Once a choice is made among the options, continuing feedback and adjustment over time may be needed (particularly in cases of chronic disease), taking into account new patient data coupled with relevant medical knowledge. These follow-up processes involve a series of choices and the exercise of judgment at each point, but judgment should be highly structured, not open-ended. That is, ongoing judgments should be structured within processes that are rigorously organized and documented (the subject of part VI below) as well as continuously informed by reliable knowledge coupling.

c. *Physician objections to separate stages of decision making*

Physicians tend to reject compartmentalizing of the decision making process into separate stages. On their view, continual exercise of informed judgment by gifted, highly trained and experienced experts is superior to a rigid combinatorial approach where pre-determined data are collected uniformly and linked to medical knowledge without resort to expert judgment. Moreover, on this view, it is an illusion to think that compartmentalizing the two stages of decision making protects against the pitfalls of human judgment. Judgment is inescapable throughout. In the first stage of decision making, preexisting medical judgments by *someone* determine what options should be considered, what counts as evidence for and against those options, and what initial data should be collected as evidence. That someone, on this view, should be the treating physician—not the patient, not third party payers, not clinical researchers, and not the authors of texts, clinical guidelines or software tools. Only the treating physician's judgment, on this view, combines medical science, firsthand contact with the individual patient, firsthand experience with similar medical problems in many other patients and the resulting intuitions. Only the treating physician has the expertise to integrate advanced medical knowledge and experience with each patient's individual needs.

This point of view overlooks the dependence of expert judgment in the second stage on information processing in the first stage. That information processing "has often acquired the pejorative label of 'just pattern recognition,'" as Dr. Geoffrey Norman has observed, "presumably because it appears to the expert to occur so rapidly and effortlessly."[96] Physicians and other experts tend to believe that they have special analytical skills going far beyond mere pattern recognition. But the evidence does not support their belief. "Studies of expertise have repeatedly demonstrated that the expert is distinguished, not by the possession of any general skills, but by the ready availability from memory of appropriate knowledge to resolve the problem. The expert is an expert primarily because he has seen it all before."[97]

Of course physician experts have *not* seen it all before. And their judgments based on whatever they may have seen before are highly fallible—even when the problem at hand is within the scope of that prior experience. The only protection from this fallibility is to compartmentalize the two stages of decision making. And the only way to do that is to rely on external tools as the first and primary vehicle for information processing. External tools directly reveal new patterns and relationships that the human mind may only infer indirectly, if at all (see part VII below). To that extent, expert judgment is superseded, just as the stethoscope is superseded for diagnosing what chest X-rays reveal directly.

In our efforts to improve decision making, the guiding principle should be to continuously improve the *basis* for decisions in the first stage as a foundation for exercising judgment in the second stage. Improving the basis for decisions not

---

96   Norman G R. Problem-solving skills, solving problems and problem-based learning. *Med Educ* 1988;22: 279-86 (p. 282).

97   *Ibid.*, p. 280

only informs the exercise of judgment but also clarifies what *kind* of judgment and *whose* judgment are relevant to the problem at hand (see part V.A.2 below for discussion of this point). Above all, improving the basis for decisions involves gathering *feedback* and acting on it over time—the key to continuous improvement of any complex activity.

In medicine, continuous improvement in the basis for decision making is not attainable unless a combinatorial approach is enabled with knowledge coupling software. Improvement may then occur at many levels, as we discuss further in part VII below.

Some physicians may choose to believe that their exceptional minds are capable of selecting and analyzing initial data as well or better than lesser minds equipped with external tools. These physicians, however, must admit that their expertise is not available to most of those who need it, nor is it transparent and subject to organized, continuous, verifiable improvement. And those physicians must admit that even their judgments may on occasion be wrong. Indeed, their exceptional ability may magnify the error. In the words of Bacon, "the very skill and swiftness of him who runs not in the right direction, must increase his aberration."[98]

Moreover, regardless of ability, a physician's personal experiences in patient care inevitably affect his or her judgments of what patient data should be collected and what the data mean. (This becomes explicit whenever physicians justify their conclusions with the statement, "in my experience ... ") Yet any physician's personal experience is inevitably limited and randomly different from that of other physicians. Judgment should be informed and tested by evidence that may lie outside personal experience and that may contradict beliefs derived from experience. Merely personal judgment should not compromise the first stage of decision making.

Enforcing this principle was the original goal of evidence-based medicine. But that goal is not achievable by evidence-based medicine in its current form. Evidence-based medicine compromises decisions by misplaced use of population-based knowledge for unique individual patients. The only way to extract some utility from population-based knowledge for patient care, and above all the only way to develop a more individualized body of medical knowledge, is to enforce detailed data collection on all patients, without the case-by-case exercise of judgment as to what initial data are necessary.

To permit judgmental departures from a combinatorial minimum standard increases each patient's exposure to wrong judgments. And a wrong judgment of initial data can be disastrous. Consider again the Addison's disease case. There, the initial data were sufficient to suggest the correct diagnosis. Yet, the

98   Aphorism No. 61 (see note 1 above).

physicians misjudged the data and thereby overlooked the correct diagnosis for months. Their patient almost died as they wandered down the various blind alleys their judgments suggested.

What is needed is a system designed to minimize erroneous judgments while incorporating prior, accurate judgments applicable to the problem at hand. This is traditionally a central function of experts—not just to exercise judgment but first to apply established knowledge. This means filtering out extraneous prior judgments and identifying relevant prior judgments for solving the problem at hand—that is, moving from the outer to the middle circle of knowledge (see part IV.F above). This research function is not feasible in settings where time is short, economic pressures are intense and information is in a state of disorder. Studies of professional expertise thus suggest that "an individual's ability to 'bring order to the informational chaos that characterizes one's everyday environment' determines whether that professional continues to perform competently."[99]

Bringing order to informational chaos is precisely what knowledge coupling software accomplishes. It does so far more efficiently than physicians could ever do. And once these basic information processing tasks are carried out, human judgment becomes far more accurate, efficient and powerful. Stated differently, the right software tools enable ordinary human judgment to *accomplish* what costly expert judgment can merely attempt.

To reiterate, judgment is empowered when (1) directly relevant information is presented in an organized form with extraneous information filtered out, and (2) time is available to consider that information with care. Knowledge coupling software is thus designed to filter and organize information, freeing up time for the practitioner and patient to consider it thoroughly. Moreover, the software incorporates pre-existing medical judgments that were reached under ideal conditions. Software builders have more opportunity than practicing physicians to exercise careful judgment (and document it) when evaluating the medical literature. The literature in turn offers peer-reviewed judgments of leading authorities who similarly have more opportunity than ordinary practitioners to deliberate with care.

In some cases, knowledge coupling software reveals a clear solution at the initial workup, with little judgment required. These cases are the low-hanging fruit. In more difficult cases, however, the initial workup reveals uncertainty and the need for follow-up investigation.

---

99   Pew Health Professions Commission, *Reforming Health Care Workforce Regulation*, San Francisco: The Commission, 1995, p. 26, quoting Pottinger, *Competence Testing As a Basis for Licensing: Problems and Prospects*, Washington, D.C., National Center for the Study of the Professions, 1977.

That investigation must be carried out in a scientifically rigorous manner. What that means is the subject of part VI below. As we shall see, just as knowledge coupling software minimizes the role of expert clinical judgment during the initial workup, so rigorous scientific practices lessen the need for expert clinical judgments during follow-up processes after the initial workup.

Before turning to follow-up processes in part VI, we further examine the notion of lessening reliance on expert judgment. This notion contradicts the expectations of highly educated people in general and physicians in particular. Advanced education teaches its recipients to rely heavily on their own minds in applying established knowledge. In no field is this more true than in medicine. Recall Dr. Nuland's words: "Our most rewarding moments of healing derive not from the works of our hearts but from those of our intellects."[100] Professional education and credentialing offer further rewards of money and status for reliance on intellect. The works of our creative intellects are indeed central to the activity of developing new knowledge. But that activity should not be the model for applying established medical knowledge. In applying knowledge, personal intellect should be subordinate to *system*; personal discipline and character and empathy should be what primarily distinguishes practitioners.

Medicine's failure to subordinate the role of intellect runs directly counter to the development of both modern science and market economies. Medicine indeed lags centuries behind those other domains, as we shall see in part V. That historical background illuminates the changes needed in medical practice, to which we will return in part VI.

---

100 See note 55 above.

V.
"Idols of the Mind": Medicine, Science, and Commerce

Medicine is built on a foundation laid by scientific knowledge. Medical *practice*, however, lacks a corresponding foundation in scientific behavior. This disparity between the behaviors of medical and scientific practitioners raises two basic questions. First, how did medical practice diverge from science in defining the behaviors expected of practitioners? Second, is it feasible to bring disciplined scientific behavior from the sheltered conditions of research to the difficult conditions of medical practice, where variables are uncontrolled and practitioners must cope with whatever problems patients present? The first question takes us back 400 years to Francis Bacon, the first thinker who systematically examined the intellectual behaviors on which modern science depends. The second question takes us from the domain of science to the domain of commerce, where scientific knowledge and technology are applied more reliably and economically than has ever been achieved in most of medical practice.

A. Medicine and the development of science

Like medicine, science has always faced a wide gap between limited human capacities and the demands of effective practice. To bridge that gap, science uses external tools such as measuring instruments, the microscope, the telescope, and the computer. The same is true of physicians and researchers in the applied science of medicine. Everything from stethoscopes to advanced imaging devices, for example, make possible clinical observations that are not otherwise within human capacity.

The tool of greatest interest for our purposes is the computer. Just as scientific instruments extend the powers of human sense organs, so the computer extends the powers of the mind. In recent decades, the mind's powers and limits have been the object of study by cognitive psychologists. Although its powers of instinctive judgment are impressive in some contexts, the mind is "a relatively inefficient device for noticing, selecting, categorizing, recording, retaining, retrieving and manipulating information for inferential purposes."[101]   Therefore, science, including medical science, has embraced modern electronic information tools:

> The dominant trend in biomedical science and in medical practice, as in every realm of science, is the increasing value and usage of computers. The data so painstakingly extracted in past years are now, through progress in biomedicine, produced in such volumes as to require computers just to record them. The scientist spends more and more time using the computer to record, analyze, compare and display their data to extract knowledge.[102]

This statement begins by equating biomedical science and medical practice. Yet, the examples given are drawn from science, not practice. Here we need to recognize two distinctions. Using the computer to extract new knowledge for medical science differs from using it to apply existing knowledge for medical practice. And, within medical practice, using the computer as a component of medical devices to enhance the user's physical capabilities differs from using it as an information tool to empower the mind for clinical decision making.

These distinctions suggest that physicians and scientists differ fundamentally in their approach to limited human capacities. Physicians recognize limits in their capacity for observation and data processing, but not in their capacity for applying medical knowledge. Thus, the most advanced, costly and ubiquitous use of computer technology in modern medicine is sophisticated clinical imaging devices. These devices collect detailed data and use sophisticated software to assemble the data into images of internal organs. By comparison, physicians rarely use computer software to assemble patient data and medical knowledge into options and evidence for medical decision making. Instead, physicians rely largely on personal intellect ("clinical judgment") for this pivotal function.

1. Intellect and the culture of science

In contrast to medical practice, science has advanced by developing alternatives to unaided judgment. These developments made possible intellectual operations that would otherwise be prohibitively laborious and prone to error. The development of mathematics, for example, was described in these terms

---

101 Grove W, Meehl P. Comparative efficiency of informal (subjective, impressionistic) and formal (mechanical, algorithmic) prediction procedures: the clinical-statistical controversy. *Psychology, Public Policy and Law* 1996; 2:293-323, p. 316, at   http://www.tc.umn.edu/~pmeehl/167GroveMeehlClinstix.pdf.

102 NIH Working Group on Biomedical Computing, *The Biomedical Information Science and Technology Initiative.* 1999. Available at http://www.nih.gov/about/director/060399.htm.

by Alfred North Whitehead. He argued that confining the role of judgment facilitates development of system or method while freeing the mind for tasks where judgment is essential. Writing of geometry before Descartes, Whitehead observed: "Every proposition has to be proved by a *fresh display of ingenuity*; and a science of which this is true lacks the great requisite of scientific thought, namely, method" (emphasis added).[103] Writing of algebra, he observed that using symbols in equations "is invariably an immense simplification," enabling "transitions in reasoning almost mechanically by the eye, which otherwise would call into play the higher faculties of the brain." Writing of arithmetic, he explained the simplifying effects of notation:

> By relieving the brain of all unnecessary work, a good notation sets it free to concentrate on more advanced problems, and in effect increases the mental power of the race. Before the introduction of the Arabic notation, multiplication was difficult, and the division even of integers called into play the highest mathematical faculties. ... Our modern power of easy reckoning with decimal fractions is the almost miraculous result of the gradual discovery of a perfect notation.

Giving these examples from mathematics, Whitehead then stated a broader principle: "It is a profoundly erroneous truism ... that we should cultivate the habit of thinking about what we are doing. The precise opposite is the case. Civilization advances by extending the number of important operations which we can perform without thinking about them."[104]

A prime example is the invention of writing. The tools and techniques of writing extend our minds to past thoughts and words without our having to

---

103 Whitehead A. *An Introduction to Mathematics*, 1911 (American ed., Oxford Univ. Press, 1948, p. 83). Whitehead's point does not apply to geometry after Descartes, who brought mathematical methods to geometry, and sought to bring analogous methods to philosophy. He wrote of the need "to avoid precipitancy and prejudice," "to comprise nothing more in my judgment than what was presented to my mind so clearly and distinctly as to exclude all ground of doubt," "to divide each of the difficulties under examination into as many parts as possible," and "to make enumerations so complete, and reviews so general, that I might be assured that nothing was omitted. The long chains of simple and easy reasonings by means of which geometers are accustomed to reach the conclusions of their most difficult demonstrations, had led me to imagine that all things, to the knowledge of which man is competent, are mutually connected in the same way ... , " *Discourse on Method*, http://www.gutenberg.org/files/59/59-h/59-h.htm. The concepts of method stated by Whitehead and Descartes are the antithesis of clinical judgment as typically exercised by physicians.

104 *An Introduction to Mathematics*, pp. 39-42. F. A. Hayek found Whitehead's principle to have profound significance in economics, as discussed in part V.B below.

recall them. Indeed, Gibbon observed that our capacity for "knowledge and reflection" depends in large part on the use of writing:

> Without that artificial help, the human memory soon dissipates or corrupts the ideas entrusted to her charge; and the noble faculties of the mind, no longer supplied with models or with materials, gradually forget their powers; the judgment becomes feeble and lethargic, the imagination languid or irregular. ...[105]

Gibbon here refers to enhancement of personal judgment and imagination. But writing also enhances the brain's capacity to recall and process complex information effectively. Tools and techniques for enhancing this capacity are crucial for purposes of both economic exchange (which may be the origin of writing, see part V.B below) and our present concern, scientific inquiry.

Information is the raw material of science. Yet, when information becomes complex, the mind is unreliable and inefficient, as cognitive psychologists have documented.[106] Moreover, normal human behaviors in using the mind lack the rigor that science demands. To overcome these limitations, scientists have developed a variety of practices. These practices include enforcing habitual use of tools and techniques to aid the mind, and simple standards of thoroughness and reliability. This discipline is essential to scientific progress:

> The dazzling achievements of Western post-Galilean science are attributable not to our having any better brains than Aristotle or Aquinas, but to the scientific method of accumulating objective knowledge. A very few strict rules (e.g. don't fake data, avoid parallax in reading a dial) but mostly rough guidelines about observing, sampling, recording, calculating and so forth sufficed to create this amazing social machine for producing valid knowledge. Scientists record observations at the time rather than rely on unaided memory. Precise instruments are substituted for the human eye, ear, nose and fingertips whenever these latter are unreliable. Powerful formalisms (trigonometry, calculus, probability theory, matrix algebra) are used to move from one set of numerical values to another.[107]

These practices introduce rigor and reliability to the raw material of science—information. This is achieved by compensating for the limited abilities and variable habits employed in measuring, recording and manipulating

---

105 Edward Gibbon, *The History of the Decline and Fall of the Roman Empire,* ch. IX; (Paris: Baudry's European Library, 1840), p. 200; available at http://books.google.com.

106 Grove and Meehl, note 101 above.

107 Grove and Meehl,. note 101 above.

information. That compensatory function also empowers the mind's creative capacities for judgment and imagination, but its first purpose is to enable trustworthy information processing.

Thus far we have discussed how tools and techniques for aiding the mind bridge the gaps between human cognitive limits and the complexity of science, between normal human behaviors and the rigorous habits of careful investigators. But there are other gaps that science must bridge: gaps between individual, subjective experience and shared, objective knowledge, between limited individual capacities and the greater capacities of social, cooperative endeavors.

How science bridges these gaps is illuminated by Karl Popper's distinctions among three different realms to which human knowledge and thought relate: the world of physical objects or states (World 1), the world of mental states or conscious experiences (World 2), and the world of the objective contents of thought, residing not just in the mind but externally in books, electronic devices, works of art and elsewhere (World 3). World 3 has objective content existing independently of the mind. Moreover, "World 3 is autonomous: in this world we can make theoretical discoveries in a similar way to that in which we can make geographical discoveries in World 1."[108] Popper's view departs from traditional epistemology. "Traditional epistemology has studied knowledge or thought in a subjective sense—in the sense of the ordinary usage of the words 'I know' or 'I am thinking.'" Popper distinguished knowledge in this subjective sense from scientific knowledge. "While knowledge in the sense of 'I know' belongs to [World 2], the world of subjects, scientific knowledge belongs to [World 3], the world of objective theories, objective problems and objective arguments."[109] Popper characterizes scientific knowledge in terms of theories, problems and arguments because scientific knowledge is conjectural and always potentially subject to refutation.

By bringing knowledge from World 2 into World 3, we create new opportunities to access knowledge, test it and apply it to human needs. Moving knowledge from World 2 to World 3 thus fosters an evolutionary process of natural selection, with errors and new knowledge coming to light.

Consider technologies like the printing press and the computer, techniques like decimal notation, and simple practices like recording data at the time of observation instead of relying on unaided memory—they are powerful because they accelerate the movement from World 2 to World 3. This movement is central to the culture of science, and to development of civilization. By moving to World

---

108 Popper, K. *Objective Knowledge: An Evolutionary Approach*. Oxford: Clarendon Press, 1972 (pp. 72, 106).

109 *Ibid.*, p. 108 (emphasis in original).

3, we become the agents of our own evolution. Physically we have changed little for millennia. Our brains are no better than Aristotle's. But new tools and new beliefs evolving in an objective, external realm have enabled science and civilization to develop.[110]

Remarkably, Francis Bacon envisioned all these dimensions of scientific culture at its birth four hundred years ago. As the first thinker who systematically examined the mind's role in the advancement of science, Bacon recognized that external aids to the mind are pivotal:

> The unassisted hand and the understanding left to itself possess little power. Effects are produced by means of instruments and helps, which the understanding requires no less than the hand ... those that are applied to the mind prompt or protect the understanding. ... The sole cause and root of almost every defect in the sciences is this, that while we falsely admire and extol the powers of the human mind, we do not search for its real helps.[111]

Bacon reacted against academic and ecclesiastical dogma, with its static dependence on the minds of ancient authorities (Aristotle in particular) and its reliance on intellect (through formal, scholastic disputation) as a sterile mode of inquiry. He became deeply skeptical of abstract thought divorced from observation and experience. The learning from experience by those engaged in commercial and practical activities enormously impressed Bacon. He also witnessed a flowering of intellectual life outside the universities. He came to view science and practical learning as cumulative, collaborative activities, anchored in experience, freed from received authority and the individual mind.[112]

Bacon saw a path that led away from the alchemy and astrology of his time and towards the remarkable advances in science and technology that have emerged over the last four hundred years. That progress has involved a symbiotic, evolving relationship among the creative minds of individuals, tools and practices for observation and experiment, social practices for systematic feedback on received knowledge, market and non-market systems for generating, disseminating and applying advances in knowledge, and finally, in recent decades, revolutionary

---

110 For further discussion, see *Knowledge Coupling*, note 2 above, pp. 4-5.

111 Bacon F. *Novum Organon* (1620), note 1 above, Aphorisms No. 2, No. 9.

112 Gaukroger S. *Francis Bacon and the Transformation of Early Modern Philosophy*. Cambridge University Press, 2001 (pp.10, 14-18); Kors A. "The New Vision of Francis Bacon," in Lecture 3 in *The Birth of the Modern Mind: The Intellectual History of the 17th and 18th Centuries* (recorded lectures from The Teaching Company).

information technologies that empower the human mind by expanding its limited capacities for raw information processing.

Analysis of the limits of the mind was central to Bacon's philosophy. Anticipating several currents of 20th century thought, he identified four "idols of the mind" that distort human thinking and perception:

- universal mental limitations "inherent in human nature";

- each person's disposition and acquired beliefs; each "has his own individual den or cavern, which intercepts and corrupts the light of nature";

- the limits of language, which "force the understanding, throw everything into confusion, and lead mankind into vain and innumerable controversies and fallacies";

- "various dogmas" in philosophy and the sciences, "which have become inveterate by tradition, implicit credence and neglect."[113]

Bacon understood that overcoming these idols of the mind is a difficult challenge for both the individual and society. "Our only remaining hope and salvation is to begin the whole labour of the mind again; not leaving it to itself, but directing it perpetually from the very first, and attaining our end as it were by mechanical aid."[114]

The vision of Bacon, together with Popper's distinction between Worlds 2 and 3, provide a useful prism for viewing the place of intellect within the culture of medical practice and the culture of science.

2. Intellect and the culture of medicine

One scholar has "compare[d] Bacon's plan to direct scientific activity by inculcating new habits in scientists with the much later reform of medical practice inaugurated by Joseph Lister in the late 1860s." Lister pioneered antisepsis in surgery, with the result that physicians and nurses became "subject to a *new and severe regimen* conducive to antiseptic conditions, a change which required a *complete change in the deportment of the surgical staff and medical staff.*"[115] Physicians did not embrace this change. Indeed, it took more than a decade for Lister's advance to become widely accepted, despite the enormous reduction in surgical mortality it made possible.[116]

---

113 Bacon F. *Novum Organon* (1620), note 1 above, Aphorisms No. 42-44.

114 Bacon F. *Novum Organon* (1620), Preface to Second Part, note 1 above.

115 Gaukroger, note 112 above, p. 13 (emphasis added).

116 See note 302 below for further discussion of the resistance Lister encountered. This was not an isolated example. Ignaz Semmelweis faced intense resistance when he demonstrated that

A modern analogue to antisepsis is use of information technology in medicine. Just as medical practitioners need to cleanse their hands, so they need to cleanse their minds. Just as antisepsis in surgery imposes a severe regimen and complete change in the deportment of practitioners, so using information technology to manage medical information effectively imposes new standards of data collection, analysis and recordkeeping, new feedback loops, and new occupational roles (the subjects of parts IV, VI, VII, and VIII). The culture of medicine resists these changes, just as it resisted the changes entailed by antisepsis.

The contrast between medicine and science is stark. Rather than resisting information technology, scientists have embraced it. The reason is that the culture of science, long before the advent of computers, had migrated from World 2 to World 3, from subjective, personal knowledge to shared, objective knowledge, embodied externally. Thus, as increasingly powerful computers became available in the second half of the 20th century, scientists were quick to take advantage of them. Doing so enabled them to easily perform calculations and data processing otherwise prohibitive for the unaided mind. In contrast, physicians are still mired in World 2. Medicine remains in denial of the problem for which computers offer a solution. The problem is that integrating clinical data with medical knowledge is too complex and time-consuming for the unaided mind. The solution is a meticulous, combinatorial matching process performed with external tools. Until the tool-driven, combinatorial alternative is experienced, the vulnerability of unaided judgment is not readily apparent.

The implication is that the culture of medicine must change fundamentally, to become more like the culture of science. At this point, however, some readers may raise two questions. First, medical practice seems to call for different forms of expertise than scientific research. Second, the purpose and context of medical practice differ radically from scientific research. We address these issues next.

a. Alternative concepts of expertise

Psychologists and philosophers distinguish between explicit knowledge (associated with conscious, deliberate analysis and judgment) and tacit knowledge (associated with intuitive or instinctive judgment), expressed in the phrases "knowing that" and "knowing how," respectively.[117] Explicit knowledge involves factual information, principles and logical relationships that can be articulated.

---

hand washing by obstetricians dramatically reduced maternal deaths in childbirth. Even now, hand washing practices are not always rigorously enforced in some contexts, despite the clear benefit to patients.

117 Barbiero, D. "Tacit knowledge." *Dictionary of Philosophy of Mind,* http://philosophy. uwaterloo.ca/MindDict/tacitknowledge.html.

Tacit knowledge involves skills and perceptions that cannot be fully articulated ("we know more than we can tell").

Science is concerned with developing explicit knowledge and thereby improving conscious, deliberate judgment. Tacit knowledge and intuitive judgment are generally considered non-scientific, although scientists often study them for purposes of developing new explicit knowledge and improving deliberate judgment. Scientists themselves use intuition to originate hypotheses, but then they test those hypotheses to arrive at explicit knowledge.

Experts other than research scientists, including professionals such as physicians, apply an amalgam of explicit and tacit knowledge. The specialized nature of this expert knowledge distinguishes these experts from the general public. A cardiac surgeon, for example, has explicit scientific knowledge about the cardiovascular system, plus tacit knowledge of (*i.e.* skill in) cardiac surgery procedures, plus further tacit knowledge growing out of personal experience with cardiac patients.

The culture of graduate medical education, medical research and much specialty care emphasizes explicit over tacit knowledge. Scientific understanding of pathophysiology is viewed as the core element of physician expertise. The acquired knowledge and analytical capacity involved in that expertise is what Sherwin Nuland described as "every doctor's measure of his own abilities ... the most important ingredient in his professional self-image" (see note 55 above). Some practitioners may view their developed intuitions (the "art of medicine") as no less important than scientific knowledge and analysis, but they still view the latter as essential to their expertise.

A competing school of thought emphasizes tacit knowledge as the basis of expertise. Indeed, expertise is sometimes *defined* as possession of specialized tacit knowledge, because experts uniquely rely on specialized tacit knowledge that cannot be communicated to others, whereas explicit knowledge within the specialty can be communicated by experts to others in textual form. This school of thought finds support in research showing the impressive powers of instinctive judgment. These powers have been studied in many contexts, not limited to professional expertise. Relying on this school of thought, Malcolm Gladwell's bestseller *Blink* argues that conscious, deliberate judgments are often less trustworthy than first impressions and snap judgments ("rapid cognition").[118] Gladwell suggests two reasons for this phenomenon. First, deliberate decision making often buries the few key factors that matter in excessive information (the needle-in-a-haystack problem). Second, deliberate decision making lacks the

---

118 Gladwell M. *Blink*, note 78, pp. 13-14.

power of our "adaptive unconscious" to comprehend intangible, unarticulated factors of relevance.

The two competing schools of thought just described both view expert judgment as resting on a set of cognitive abilities (knowledge, analytical skill and intuition) that only experts can acquire and apply. A completely different school of thought points in a different direction. This school discounts the value of expert decision making, regardless of whether expertise is attributed to deliberate or instinctive judgment. As summarized by professors William Grove and Paul Meehl, decades of studies in various fields (including medicine) have compared subjective, impressionistic, expert judgments with mechanical, algorithmic procedures such as multiple regression, weighted sums of predictive factors, and actuarial tables. These procedures combine items of data (*e.g.* findings on a patient) to arrive at predictive conclusions (*e.g.* diagnoses) in a formulaic manner. Grove and Meehl conclude that the mechanical procedures perform as well or marginally better than the judgments of expensive expert professionals. Other cognitive psychologists have reached similar conclusions. "In fact, there is even evidence that when [mechanical] aids are offered, many experts attempt to improve upon these aids' predictions—and they do worse than they would have had they "mindlessly" adhered to them."[119] Based on such evidence, Grove and Meehl argue that the legal authority conferred on expensive experts in many contexts is not justified.[120] In terms of the two stages of medical decision making discussed in part IV.G.5 above, this school of thought suggests that human judgment should be minimized not only in the first stage of decision making, as argued here, but also in the second stage, contrary to what is argued here.

To summarize the above discussion, we have identified three alternative bases for expert decisions—(1) deliberate judgments based on explicit knowledge, (2) instinctive judgments based on tacit knowledge, and (3) mechanical substitutes for judgment—plus three schools of thought about these alternatives. The prevailing school of thought in science and academic medicine is that deliberate judgment is primary. The second school of thought, accepted by many medical practitioners, is that the power of instinctive judgment is undervalued and deserves increased acceptance. The third school of thought, accepted by many cognitive psychologists, is that both deliberate and instinctive judgments

---

119 Dawes R. *Rational Choice in an Uncertain World* (New York: Harcourt Brace Jovanovich, Inc. 1988), p. 143.

120 Grove W, Meehl P. Comparative efficiency of informal (subjective, impressionistic) and formal (mechanical, algorithmic) prediction procedures: the clinical-statistical controversy. *Psychology, Public Policy and Law* 1996; 2:293-323, p. 316. See also Dawes R. *Rational Choice in an Uncertain World*, pp. 202-19.

are overvalued and very often should be replaced with formulaic, non-judgmental alternatives.

All three of these schools of thought fail to distinguish between the two stages of medical decision making. Recall that the first stage involves raw information processing; the second stage involves the exercise of judgment. In the first stage, the mind's weaknesses cripple the information processing on which judgment depends. Thus, all forms of human judgment and substitutes for judgment are unreliable in the second stage of decision making, because important information is so often overlooked in the first stage. That explains why the studies cited by Grove and Meehl show the accuracy of human judgment to be only marginally different from non-judgmental substitutes, and why both are highly fallible. Their fallibility diminishes, however, when external tools and standards of care are used to assemble information in the first stage of decision making.

This is the reality that Francis Bacon understood four centuries ago. One century ago Dr. William Osler recognized this same reality when he observed:

> Books are tools, doctors are craftsmen, and so truly as one can measure the development of any particular handicraft by the variety and complexity of its tools, so we have no better means of judging the intelligence of a profession than by its general collection of books. A physician who does not use books and journals, who does not need a library, who does not read one or two of the best weeklies and monthlies, soon sinks to the level of the cross-counter prescriber, and not alone in practice, but in those mercenary feelings and habits which characterize a trade."[121]

Now Osler would say that a physician who does not use external information tools to apply knowledge from books and journals soon sinks to the level of an amateur, losing the status of a scientific expert. "It is astonishing with how little reading a doctor can practice medicine, but it is not astonishing how badly he can do it," Osler said. Osler would recognize that knowledge coupling tools are more powerful than books and journals. The tools do not depend on variable physician behaviors in recalling their own knowledge, consulting the literature for more knowledge and coupling all with patient data. This is a burden that physicians cannot be counted on to assume.[122] What is needed is an enforceable system of care that does not rely on what the doctor unilaterally does.

---

121 Quoted in Cushing H. *The Life of Sir William Osler* (Oxford, Clarendon Press, 1926), Vol. I, p. 448.

122 *Ibid.*, p. 345.

Here we return to the point we asserted in the preceding section—that the culture of science should govern intellectual behavior in the first stage of medical decision making. That point holds whatever the relative merits of deliberate judgment, instinctive judgment or some mechanical alternative to judgment.

This point may be hard to accept for those who believe that expertise resides primarily in tacit knowledge and instinctive judgment (a view that seems more plausible now that information technology has made specialized explicit knowledge available to non-experts). Here, we should return to Malcolm Gladwell's defense of instinctive judgment (discussed at note 78 above). Gladwell's defense misses two crucial factors. First, in arguing that instinctive judgment is better than deliberate judgment at finding the needle buried in a haystack of detailed information, he overlooks that information technology is fast enough to search the entire haystack without resorting to judgmental guesswork. Second, in arguing that our "adaptive unconscious" is often more effective than conscious deliberate judgment, he overlooks the weakness of *both* forms of judgment, relative to external tools.

Many physicians recognize that instinctive judgment is not to be trusted. They put their faith in deliberate judgment based on explicit, scientific knowledge, as we have discussed. Indeed, this point of view underlies both the patient safety movement and the demand for evidence-based medicine.

The patient safety movement has brought new attention to decades of research in cognitive psychology. Rediscovering Bacon's first "idol of the mind" (see note 113 above), that research has shown us again how the mind's normal propensities lead it into error. These insights from cognitive psychology influenced clinicians such as Lucian Leape, whose "Error in Medicine"[123] argued that medical error contributes to an epidemic of iatrogenic illness and injury. Public awareness of this epidemic has increased. But awareness alone is not enough to bring about change. Moreover, awareness has focused on failures of execution, not decision making (see note 36 above). Failures of decision making are more difficult to confront, in part because correcting them demands change in the foundations of medical practice. And change at that level increases the threat to the status quo. The status quo is insulated from accountability and competition that might otherwise bring about sustainable change (see parts V.B and VIII.B below).

Some readers may question whether standards of intellectual behavior from the culture of science can apply in the culture of medicine, because there are fundamental differences between those two domains. But the differences only heighten the need to introduce disciplined scientific behaviors.

---

123 Leape L. Error in Medicine. *JAMA* 1994; 272:1851-1857.

b. Comparing scientific research and medical practice

In comparison with scientific research (Bacon's concern), medical decision making is even more vulnerable to the universal mental weaknesses that Bacon identified and cognitive psychology has studied. Medicine involves human situations where personal experience makes indelible impressions (for example, a physician who saves a patient's life with a chosen therapy and then uncritically uses that therapy with other patients for whom it may not be the best option). At the same time, medicine involves a vast body of knowledge that is at once too complex for anyone to fully comprehend and yet not complex enough to fully capture the realities of individual patients. Practitioners under severe time pressures apply whatever knowledge enters the mind at the point of care. Often that is not the precise knowledge most applicable to the unique patient but rather fragments of personal knowledge and beliefs evoked in the physician's mind by limited data. In Bacon's words:

> The human understanding is most excited by that which strikes and enters the mind at once and suddenly, and by which the imagination is immediately filled and excited. It then begins almost imperceptibly to conceive and suppose that every-thing is similar to the few objects which have taken possession of the mind; while it is very slow and unfit for the transition to the remote and heterogeneous instances by which axioms are tried by fire, unless the office be imposed upon it by severe regulations, and a powerful authority.[124]

It might seem that enforcing "evidence-based medicine" provides the "severe regulation" and "powerful authority" needed to break the hold of personal experience on judgment. But evidence-based medicine in its present form is "slow and unfit" to move from the population-based generalizations of medical knowledge to "the remote and heterogeneous instances" of unique patients (see part VII below). Moreover, evidence-based medicine leaves unsolved the needle-in-a-haystack problem—the difficulty of coupling vast knowledge with detailed data to find the crucial combinations of details relevant to an individual patient.

In contrast to evidence-based medicine, the combinatorial approach solves the needle-in-a-haystack problem. It does so by enforcing use of external tools to collect and process detailed data, without error and omission. In this way, the combinatorial approach provides the "severe regulations" and "powerful authority" that Bacon called for. Scientifically, two crucial benefits result. First, the combinatorial approach generates multiple hypotheses, that is, the full

---

124 Bacon F. *Novum Organon* (1620), note 1 above, Aphorism No. 47.

range of diagnostic or therapeutic possibilities suggested by detailed findings on a patient.[125] Second, those possibilities include Bacon's "heterogeneous instances" that may contradict a favored diagnostic or therapeutic hypothesis. In both these ways, the combinatorial approach enforces scientific "trial by fire," going beyond the mind's normal propensities.

The need for external aids to the mind is only reinforced when we further compare science and medical practice. Scientists and practicing physicians engage in fundamentally different problem solving activities, in terms of both purpose and context. First, in terms of purpose, as Chris Weed has observed[126], scientists seek to *discover* knowledge while practitioners seek to *use* established knowledge for solving more-or-less familiar problems. Although each patient is unique, patient problems are sufficiently familiar so that established knowledge can often be applied effectively. Unfamiliar problems may arise that are truly inconsistent with or unencompassed by established knowledge. But practicing

---

125 The systematic practice of generating multiple hypotheses has been characterized as an "intellectual invention ... needed to round out the Baconian scheme" of inductive inference. Platt J. Science, Strong Inference – Proper Scientific Method (The New Baconians), *Science* 146:3642; 347-353 (Oct. 16, 1964), available in full text at http://256.com/gray/docs/strong_inference.html. Inquiring why fields of science vary in their productivity, this article attributes higher productivity in some fields to a culture of rapidly seeking and testing multiple hypotheses. This contrasts with a "more relaxed and diffuse tradition" of focusing on one hypothesis at a time, which leads to a tendency to "do busywork," and "become 'method- oriented' rather than 'problem-oriented.'" Quoting an earlier article (that echoes Bacon), this article explains: "'The moment one has offered an original explanation for a phenomenon which seems satisfactory, that moment affection for his intellectual child springs into existence ... There springs up also unwittingly a pressing of the theory to make it fit the facts and a pressing of the facts to make them fit the theory... To avoid this grave danger, the method of multiple working hypotheses is urged. It differs from the simple working hypothesis in that it distributes the effort and divides the affections. .... Each hypothesis suggests its own criteria, its own method of proof, its own method of developing the truth, and if a group of hypotheses encompass the subject on all sides, the total outcome of means and of methods is full and rich.'"

In addition to these benefits at the individual level, generating multiple hypotheses has benefits at the social level: "The conflict and exclusion of alternatives that is necessary to sharp inductive inference has been all too often a conflict between men, each with his single Ruling Theory. But whenever each man begins to have multiple working hypotheses, it becomes purely a conflict between ideas. It becomes much easier then for each of us to aim every day at conclusive disproofs - at strong inference - without either reluctance or combativeness." In medicine, physicians tend to become wedded to a narrow range of hypotheses based on specialty orientation, financial considerations, time pressures and personal pride. That narrow approach is inefficient and prone to error, as illustrated by the diffuse, aimless diagnostic attempts in the Addison's disease case study (part II.A above). These tendencies can be overcome by moving from Popper's World 2 to World 3, using external tools to generate multiple hypotheses and the evidence to test them.

126 C.C. Weed. The Philosophy, Use and Interpretation of Knowledge Couplers, note 2 above, p. 1.

physicians are not expected to develop new knowledge about these truly unfamiliar situations. Instead, physicians seek to apply established knowledge as well as possible to situations that resemble prior practice.

Second, turning from purpose to context, the contexts in which scientists and physicians act are fundamentally different. Research environments shelter scientists from difficulties that practitioners must cope with on a daily basis. Scientists choose the problems to investigate, they have the time and resources to pursue those problems in depth, and they create controlled conditions needed to isolate and understand relevant variables. Scientists thus work under ideal conditions for human judgment. In contrast, practicing physicians must function without the luxuries of choice, ample time, sufficient resources and controlled conditions. Physicians may not choose which patients they wish to care for, nor which patient problems they wish to investigate. Physicians may devote only limited time and financial resources to each patient, in comparison to what scientists may devote to their investigations. And physicians have little opportunity to create controlled conditions for isolating variables of interest. On the contrary, physicians must care for complex patients with multiple interacting variables over time. Each patient thus represents a unique combination of variables. That individuality demands rapidly processing an enormous volume of information and then following through in a highly organized manner over time.

These differences in purpose and context mean that the need for external tools and standards is greater, not less, in medical practice than in scientific research. There is no other way of matching established knowledge with patients' medical situations (part IV) or organizing the total processes of care (part VI).

These conclusions are consistent with the school of thought in cognitive psychology that discounts the value of expert judgment (recall our discussion at notes 119 - 120). Yet, this school of thought has had little effect on the marketplace for expert judgment, in medicine or elsewhere. The psychologist Robyn Dawes, referring to Professor Meehl (see note 120), attributes this state of affairs in part to social, economic and legal factors:

What effect have these findings had on the *practice* of expert judgment? Almost zilch. Meehl was elected president of the American Psychological Association at a strikingly young age, and the implications of his work were ignored by his fellow psychologists. States license psychologists, physicians and psychiatrists to make (lucrative) global judgments of the form "It is my opinion that ..." [P]eople have great misplaced confidence in their global judgments, a confidence that is strong enough to dismiss an impressive body of research findings and to find its way into the legal system.[127]

Dawes further explains that this state of affairs also reflects emotional needs:

> The greatest obstacle to using [external aids] may be the difficulty of convincing ourselves that we should take precautions against ourselves ...
> . Most of us ... seek to maximize our flexibility of judgment (and power). The idea that a self-imposed external constraint on action can actually enhance our freedom by releasing us from predictable and undesirable *internal* constraints is not a popular one. ... The idea that such internal constraints can be cognitive, as well as emotional, is even less palatable.[128]

In its differences from the domain of science, medicine resembles the domain of commerce. Comparing science and commerce in relation to medicine is important, because medical care must be provided efficiently, without unnecessary use of scarce resources, regardless of whether the setting is commercial or non-profit.

B. Economy of knowledge in decision making

1. *The domain of commerce*

Commercial enterprises, more so than research enterprises, must cope with the ongoing costs of gaining information resources and engaging in decision processes. Although often overlooked, the economic importance of these costs, as Thomas Sowell observes, is fundamental:

> In reality, knowledge can be enormously costly, and is often scattered in uneven fragments, too small to be individually usable in decision making. The communication and coordination of these scattered fragments of knowledge is one of the basic problems—perhaps *the* basic problem—of any society, as well as its constituent institutions and relationships.[129]

---

127 Dawes R. *Rational Choice in an Uncertain World* (New York: Harcourt Brace Jovanovich, Inc. 1988), p. 208 (emphasis in original). The term "global judgment" refers to an intuitive judgment about a complex, multivariate situation as a whole, where the judgment is made without separately weighing the pro and con factors. Research shows that judgments based on a weighted average of pro and con factors, where the weighting of each factor is intuitive, are consistently superior to intuitive *global* judgments. *Ibid.*, pp. 202-03.

128 *Ibid.*, p. 143 (emphasis in original).

129 Sowell T. *Knowledge and Decisions.* New York: Basic Books, 1980, p. 26. Sowell makes this point in the context of arguing that informal relationships can be more efficient and effective than formal organizations in communicating, coordinating and applying scattered fragments of knowledge. Our point is that both formal organizations and informal relationships depend on

Solving this basic problem in most contexts requires (1) recordkeeping *devices* external to the mind; and (2) recordkeeping *standards* enabling the devices to communicate information. Together, these two elements move information from Popper's World 2 to World 3. For example, paper and ink are recordkeeping devices; alphabets and numerals for writing are recordkeeping standards. These ancient innovations appear to have originated for purposes of economic exchange (although writing evolved to serve additional purposes). Ultimately, transactional recordkeeping evolved into double-entry accounting standards that permitted economic exchange of much greater scale and complexity than was previously possible.[130] Indeed, scholars conjecture that double-entry bookkeeping was essential to the development of capitalism, with its "invisible hand" and spontaneous order.[131] Accounting "'makes success and failure, profit and loss ascertainable. ... Our civilization is inseparably linked with our methods of economic calculation. It would perish if we were to abandon this most precious intellectual tool of acting.'"[132]

These points lead to the issue of recordkeeping devices and standards in medicine. The issue is quite different for medicine than for many commercial enterprises. The goal in many enterprises is to achieve uniformity of outputs by eliminating variation of inputs. The goal of medical decision making is just the opposite—to individualize care by taking variation into account. One central difficulty in achieving this goal is that medical knowledge is usually expressed as generalizations that fit unique patients imperfectly. Those generalizations are

moving knowledge from Popper's World 2 to World 3. See our discussion at note 108 above.

130 "Humans have created and stored transactional records outside their brains for at least 10,000 years. Archeologists have discovered nonwritten transactional artifacts that date to 8,000 BCE and have documented that the independent invention of writing by the Sumerians (ca 3,200 BCE) was for keeping records. Both of these innovations appeared concurrently with scale expansions in human settlements. Anthropologists demonstrate that symbolic artifacts serving a memory function are often a central feature of complex exchange in primitive societies. Scholars have suggested that the recordkeeping of modern accounting provides just such a memory aid." Basu S. et al., Recordkeeping alters economic history by promoting reciprocity. *Proceedings of the National Academy of Sciences.* 106:1009-1014 (Jan. 27, 2009), p. 1009 (citations omitted), available at http://www.pnas.org/content/106/4/1009.full. This article presents experimental evidence from a market simulation designed to test how recordkeeping alters economic behaviors.

131 Waymire G, Basu S. *Accounting is an Evolved Economic Institution.* Emory University School of Law, Law and Economics Research Paper Series No. 08-33 (2008), pp. 11, 87-93. Available at http://papers.ssrn.com/sol3/papers.cfm?abstract_id=1155420)

132 *Ibid.,* p. 88, quoting Ludwig Mises. Waymire and Basu go on to discuss the "links between double entry accounting, human cognition and organizational form and performance." The linkage is essentially that "accounting systems construct the information (from raw transactional data) that fuels the search for comparative advantage by the modern corporation ..." *Ibid.,* pp. 88, 91.

essential to take into account but cannot properly be applied without also taking into account detailed, patient-specific data *and* individual preferences or values of each patient. These disparate elements must be combined for individualized decisions, but those involved in medical decisions are not positioned to do so on their own. Practitioners cannot judge how patients' personal preferences or values should be applied. Nor are either patients or practitioners able to efficiently mobilize relevant general knowledge or couple that knowledge with detailed data. Thus, the dilemma presented by medical decision making is to enable the parties involved to take into account information too complex for them to process on their own.

This dilemma exists and is resolved to varying degrees in many economic contexts. To understand how it is resolved, recall Whitehead's principle—"civilization advances by extending the number of important operations which we can perform without thinking about them." F. A. Hayek found Whitehead's principle to have "profound significance in the social field." Its significance lies in economy of knowledge:

> We make constant use of formulas, symbols and rules whose meaning we do not understand and through the use of which *we avail ourselves of the assistance of knowledge which individually we do not possess.* We have developed these practices and institutions by building upon habits and institutions which have proved successful in their own sphere and which have in turn become the foundation of the civilization we have built up.[133]

Hayek's concern was "the price system as a mechanism for communicating information." He critiqued formal equilibrium analysis in economics, which assumed away the need for such a mechanism: "there is something fundamentally wrong with an approach which habitually disregards an essential part of the phenomena with which we have to deal: the unavoidable imperfection of man's knowledge and *the consequent need for a process by which knowledge is constantly communicated and acquired*" (emphasis added). He also critiqued central planning as an inadequate process for this purpose. The price system provides an alternative to central planning. In contrast to centrally planned systems,

> the most significant fact about this [price] system is the *economy of knowledge* with which it operates, or *how little the individual participants need to know* in order to be able to take the right action. In abbreviated form, by

---

133 F.A. Hayek, "The Use of Knowledge in Society," American Economic Review, XXXV, No. 4, Sep. 1945, pp. 519-30 at p. 525 (emphasis added).

a kind of symbol, *only the most essential information is passed on and passed on only to those concerned.*[134]

The planners of a command and control economy are unable to apply their knowledge (statistical information) effectively because they are too isolated from practical knowledge of "the particular circumstances of time and place," Hayek argues. This practical knowledge "by its nature cannot enter into statistics and therefore cannot be conveyed to any central authority in statistical form. The statistics which such a central authority would have to use would have to be arrived at precisely by abstracting from minor differences between the things, ... which may be very significant for the specific decision." That practical knowledge of "minor differences" is only available to the "man on the spot" who is closest to the subject matter of the decision. "But the 'man on the spot' cannot decide solely on the basis of his limited but intimate knowledge of the facts of his immediate surroundings. There still remains the problem of communicating to him such further information as he needs to fit his decisions into the whole pattern of changes in the larger economic system."[135]   This is what the pricing system accomplishes. The pricing system is powerful, because it communicates not only information (e.g., about scarcity) but also incentives to act on that information.[136]

2. *Comparing commerce and medicine*

Just as market economies need a price system to efficiently communicate the limited information essential for individual transactions, so patients and practitioners need an efficient system for accessing and processing the limited, personalized information relevant to solving individual patient problems. Like price information, personalized medical information creates stronger market incentives than general knowledge by facilitating accurate decision making on issues of personal importance.

But personalized information is a needle in the haystack of medical knowledge and data. Patients thus face enormous uncertainty unless and until they can access the limited information relevant to their individual problems. Resolving this uncertainty for patients is the traditional role of physician experts.[137]

134 *Ibid.* at 522.

135 I*bid.* at 518.

136 Sowell T. *Knowledge and Decisions*, note 129 above, pp. 38, 167-68, and the 1996 Preface, p. xiv.

137 Arrow K. Uncertainty and the Welfare Economics of Medical Care. *American Economic Review*. 1963. LIII:941-73. For further discussion of Arrow's classic article in relation to Thomas Sowell's analysis of knowledge and decision making, see "Opening the black box of clinical judgment," note 2 above, Part IV.B, pp. 5-8.

But consumer dependence on costly experts for personal decisions interferes with the market, blocking the efficiencies that market forces otherwise tend to achieve. And market forces would respond to economic reality—the value offered by external tools. The right tools are more efficient and effective than the minds of experts for accessing the limited information relevant to unique individual problem situations.

In many economic contexts other than health care, we take for granted that personal consumption decisions do not require costly expert advice. One need not hire an engineer to buy a car; one need not hire a professional guide to determine the route for driving through unfamiliar area. Market and regulatory forces have developed systems enabling consumers to function autonomously in such contexts. Rather than rely on third party agents to make group decisions, consumers act autonomously to make individualized decisions. As Regina Herzlinger observes: "The Achilles heel of group purchasing is that it inhibits product differentiation. The fundamental principle of a market-based economy is that competition among differentiated products is much more effective in controlling costs than the clout of group purchases."[138] Differentiation, however, increases the complexity of choice for consumers. Therefore, an essential element of competition in medicine is information tools enabling consumers to cope with complexity.

In medicine, tools for reliably processing complex information can *simplify* the ultimate choices presented to consumers by filtering out what is extraneous while presenting individually relevant options and the pros and cons of each.[139] Without a system for accessing that information as needed, patients will continue to rely on the apparent expertise of practitioners. In turn, as Chris Weed has written,

> practitioners might just as well continue to rely on their own creative intuition, experience, and random and informal contacts with other concerned people. Without the routine use of powerful knowledge coupling tools to generate specific linkages of the knowledge base to practical decision-making for unique individuals, scientific medicine affects practice primarily through new procedures and associated technologies, while the application of such procedures and technologies is left to a sort of cottage industry or folk art based on something approaching oral tradition."[140]

---

138 Herzlinger, R. *Who Killed Health Care: America's $2 Trillion Health Problem and the Consumer-Driven Cure* (New York: McGraw Hill, 2007), p. 185

139 "Opening the black box of clinical judgment," note 2 above, Part IV, pp. 7-8.

140 Weed CC. "Overview," in *Knowledge Coupling*, note 2 above, p. xviii-xix.

Practitioners need knowledge coupling tools to inform their use of advanced procedures and technologies at two levels. First, in order to determine when an advanced procedure or technology is superior to other options, practitioners and patients need to elicit all relevant options, and the pros and cons of each, for that patient's specific problem situation. Second, if an advanced procedure or technology is determined to be the superior option, using it effectively may itself require careful information processing. Use of imaging technology, for example, requires taking into account a bewildering array of factors in judging alternative tests, test protocols, test limitations and the significance of test results.[141] Practitioners thus need information tools to use clinical imaging tools cost-effectively no less than they need the imaging tools themselves to reveal internal organs. In both contexts, ignoring modern technology is unacceptable.

In addition to imaging technologies, another example of problematic medical intervention is use of drug therapy. Medical decision making on drug use is fraught with complexity and peril:

> Our pharmaceutical habits today might actually make pharmacotherapy more risky than it was when all we had were herbal remedies and liquefied tree bark…. doctors today use an increasing number of drugs in combinations, and more drugs are being used more often by older people, a group that is likely to recognize fewer of the benefits of some medicines and more of their side effects. All of these trends are likely to continue to make adverse drug reactions more prevalent and profound and our efforts to mitigate them even more difficult.[142]

The difficulties make it critical to weigh drug therapies against other therapeutic alternatives, to keep track of the drugs patients are already taking, to take into account the patient's medical problems other than the problem for which the drug is prescribed, to anticipate side effects and interactions with other medical interventions, to carefully select physiological parameters for monitoring, and to meticulously collect and analyze the relevant data, including the patient's subjective responses. These demands can be met only with external tools for processing information and organizing patient data (the subjects of parts IV and VI).

---

141 Mendelson M., Murray, P. Towards the appropriate use of diagnostic imaging, *Medical Journal of Australia* 2007; 187 (1): 5-6, at http://www.mja.com.au/public/issues/187_01_020707/men10331_fm.html. This editorial argues that guidance on imaging technology needs to be in electronic form, continuously updated and integrated with other computerized systems.

142 Gottlieb S. Opening Pandora's Pillbox: Using Modern Information Tools To Improve Drug Safety. Health Affairs, July/August 2005. DOI 10.1377/hlthaff.24.4.938, pp. 938.

An unaided judgmental approach to the first stage of decision making gives practitioners free rein to use new procedures, drugs and technologies in accordance with their own intellectual and financial interests, and free rein to impose their judgments without regard to applicable knowledge. Similarly, vendors have free rein to market new technologies aggressively. Reinforcing this effect are practitioners relationships: "the current culture of medicine fosters lucrative networks of referrals and procedures but discourages critical examination of their value."[143] These elements have led analysts to conclude that technological advances (not an aging population) are the primary contributor to excess cost growth in health care.[144]

Technological innovation might have exactly the opposite effect if an objective, transparent, combinatorial approach to data collection and analysis were employed. Patients and practitioners would be equipped to critically examine the value of expensive new technologies and choose them only when superior to existing alternatives, based on each patient's individual needs in the specific problem situation. In that environment, new medical technologies could become a source of cost *decreases*—which is the role that technological advance often plays in other sectors of the economy.

3. The need for simple rules to manage complex information

Both practitioners and consumers are unable to cope with complexity when left to their own devices. Both practitioners and consumers need to rely on external systems to manage information for decision making. Moreover, they need to use these systems jointly. These systems must therefore be simple to use for everyone involved. Indeed, simplicity at the consumer level is characteristic of much economic activity outside of health care. "The growing complexity of science, technology and organization does not imply either a growing knowledge or a growing need for knowledge in the general population," as Thomas Sowell has written. "On the contrary, the increasingly complex *processes* tend to lead to increasingly simple and easily understood products. … Organizational progress parallels that in science and technology, permitting ultimate simplicity through intermediate complexity."[145] From this point of view, the health care system's impenetrable complexity is anomalous.

---

143 Groopman, J., *How Doctors Think*, note 11 above, p. 228. Physicians are powerless to resist these pressures, because their patients will simply find other physicians who act with less restraint. *Ibid.*; Jauhar, S., "Many Doctors, Many Tests, No Rhyme or Reason," note 23 above.

144 Congressional Budget Office. *The Long-Term Outlook for Health Care Spending*, March 2008, p. 6.

145 *Knowledge and Decisions*, note 129 above, pp. 10-11.

Analysis by the Institute of Medicine (IOM) points in the same direction—simplicity must be built into the health care system for patients and practitioners. The IOM cites a theoretical basis for this conclusion in the study of "complex adaptive systems." Occurring in various social and natural contexts, complex adaptive systems are not built according to external, pre-conceived designs. Rather, complex systems "can emerge from *a few simple rules* that are locally applied" by individual participants in the system (emphasis added). "It is liberating to realize that the task of complex system design does not itself need to be complex." To design an effective complex system means to "create the conditions for self-organization through simple rules under which massive and diverse experimentation can happen."[146] Based on these scientific insights, the IOM has concluded that "important lessons about simple rules for complex adaptive systems can be applied to health care systems as well. In redesigning health care, the building blocks are simple processes that make up the work of small systems of care and their interconnections."[147] The IOM proceeds to formulate "Ten Simple Rules for the 21st Century Health Care System" (pp. 70-88), but these are in reality general goals, not specific, operational rules for achieving the goals.

What are the "simple rules" needed by the health care system? A basic reality of health care is its information-intensive nature. That reality suggests that simple rules for managing complex clinical information are pivotal. Consider an analogy from the domain of commerce: accounting rules for managing complex financial information.

At first glance, accounting rules may seem like an unfortunate analogy. Complexity, not simplicity, is what most of us associate with financial accounting. Moreover, accounting rules have been powerless to prevent either the financial scandals that occurred at the beginning of this decade in cases like Enron and Worldcom, or the financial crisis that occurred near the end of the decade. Yet, the analogy with accounting reveals much about the health care system.

Accounting rules are indeed complex. But that complexity exists only at the margin. The core concepts of double-entry bookkeeping are so simple that they are taken for granted. They apply universally, and yet allow for enormous diversity. They help to organize the economic relationships among individuals who may or may not have any awareness of them. First codified in Renaissance Italy 500 years ago, the core concepts of double-entry bookkeeping still provide

---

146 IOM, *Crossing the Quality Chasm* (Washington: National Academies Press, 2001), Appendix B, Paul Plsek, "Redesigning Health Care with Insights from the Science of Complex Adaptive Systems," pp. 313, 316, available at http://books.nap.edu/openbook.php?record_id=10027.

147 IOM, *Crossing the Quality Chasm*," p. 65.

a foundation for commerce.[148] On this foundation have been built "generally accepted accounting principles" (GAAP) in the U.S. and similar standards in other countries. Accounting principles evolved spontaneously before formal standards setting, and they are generally accepted for internal use, not simply imposed as an external compliance obligation.[149] This general acceptance results from the order, transparency, feedback and accountability they make possible. To secure these benefits, private sector organizations codify and refine accounting standards, governments incorporate them in regulation, and the accounting profession is employed to enforce them with periodic audits.

The profound social and economic importance of accounting standards became obvious twice in the last decade. In cases like Enron and Worldcom, egregious accounting violations caused a major upheaval. In the recent financial crisis, financial risks were magnified, concentrated and obscured in unprecedented ways. Financial accounting standards then could not be relied upon to maintain order and transparency. Thus, the scandal was that generally accepted accounting standards were violated or allowed to become ineffective. By comparison, in health care the scandal is that generally accepted standards to manage clinical information do not even exist.

Resistance to financial accounting standards is a quite universal phenomenon. The historian Jacob Soll has described examples from five centuries. For governments, businesses, and households alike, it is difficult to follow the disciplines and face the results of financial accounting. Avoidance, "the tranquilizing effect of not knowing," is a constant threat.[150] The two major breakdowns in corporate accounting standards within the last decade show the magnitude of that threat. From this perspective, the general acceptance and enforcement of accounting standards in the domain of commerce is a remarkable, and fragile, achievement.

A comparable achievement in medicine will not come easily. But its rewards could be great. We have discussed how double-entry accounting standards enabled economic development of a scale and complexity not otherwise possible (see notes 130 - 132 above). We cannot know whether comparable advances in medicine would result from enforcing rigorous standards of care for managing clinical information. Regardless, applying these standards offers more immediate

---

148 http://en.wikipedia.org/wiki/Double_entry_bookkeeping.

149 See Waymire and Basu, note 131 above.

150 Soll J. "Avoidance by the Numbers," New York *Times*, Nov. 21, 2009, http://www.nytimes.com/2009/11/22/opinion/22soll.html?adxnnl=1&adxnnlx=1258931125-Zu0ZwcxfMLMLKqx-U7TtI5w.

and personal rewards for practitioners. Professor Soll, giving an example outside of medicine from the 17th Century, suggests one aspect of those rewards:

> Samuel Pepys, the secretary to the British Admiralty, wrote his famous diary every day while at the same sitting balancing his personal and state account books. They were related activities of the reckoning of each day, and Pepys, who regarded those who did not keep their own books as madmen, found catharsis in this virtuous and disciplined activity.[151]

By comparison, information management by clinicians is not cathartic but corrosive.

In part IV we focused on standards for managing clinical information at the threshold stage—the initial workup. Now we turn to standards of care for the follow-up stage, where medical records are pivotal. Bringing scientific rigor, order and transparency to medical records is no less important and no less achievable than doing so with the initial workup.

---

151 *Ibid.* See also Professor Soll's forthcoming, *The Age of Reckoning: A History of Accounting and the Problem of the Modern Age.*

VI.
Building on the Foundation: The Medical Record

A. The nature of complex cases

For some medical problems, if the right patient data are coupled with the right medical knowledge, a correct diagnosis and treatment may be immediately revealed. For other problems, however, knowledge coupling reveals numerous diagnostic or treatment options worth considering. Selecting the best option may require substantial further investigation, sometimes involving trial and error with careful monitoring over time. This is especially likely for patients with a chronic illness. Managing chronic illness often involves multiple interventions that are adjusted over time, rather than a single treatment that reaches completion.

The difficulty of handling a single complex problem escalates when patients have multiple problems. Multiple problems are characteristic of high-cost populations—older patients and those with chronic illness.[152] Their problems, and the medical interventions for each, frequently interact. The interactions can easily derail what might otherwise be well-conceived plans for each problem considered in isolation. Heightening the difficulty is that multiple problems are rarely confined to one medical specialty. No single physician is likely to have the personal expertise needed to care for a patient with multiple problems.

Another difficulty in complex cases is the limitations of medical knowledge. Medical knowledge is expressed in generalizations that at best only approximate, and often distort or hide, the realities of unique, individual patients. This gap between what physicians are educated to expect and what they actually encounter—between "knowledge" and reality—is central to the care of complex patients. Somehow, patient care must be managed in a way that comprehends both general knowledge and patient individuality. Yet, the mind's natural propensities, as described by Francis Bacon, tend to block comprehension.

---

152 IOM, *Crossing the Quality Chasm*, note 146 above, p. 27: "About 44 percent of those with a chronic illness have more than one such condition, and the likelihood of having two or more chronic conditions increases steadily with age." The IOM goes on to cite data that annual medical costs for those with more than one chronic condition are 2½ times as high as the costs for those with one chronic condition, which in turn are more than twice as high as the cost of those with acute conditions only. *Ibid.*

Beyond these analytical difficulties, complex cases present two logistical difficulties. First, numerous physiological variables and medical interventions must be tracked over time, usually over a period of years when chronic illness is involved. "The volume of data on a chronic patient becomes so large that it becomes unmanageable, and therefore lost, just as the volume of data in the medical literature is already unmanageable and lost to the average practitioner," as Dr. Ken Bartholomew has observed.[153]

The second logistical difficulty in complex cases is the need for coordination of care among multiple practitioners at multiple sites over time, while communicating with the patient throughout. Again, this difficulty is central to care of chronic disease. As described by the Institute of Medicine:

> Unlike much acute, episodic care, effective care of the chronically ill is a collaborative process, involving the definition of clinical problems in terms that both patients and providers understand; joint development of a care plan with goals, targets and implementation strategies; provision of self-management training and support services; and active, sustained follow-up using visits, telephone calls, e-mails, and Web-based monitoring and decision support programs. Much of the care provided to the chronically ill is given by patients and their families."[154]

As this description suggests, the need for collaboration implicates not only practitioners but the patient. In chronic illness, enabling patient awareness, participation and commitment is fundamental. Unavoidable complexity must somehow be made manageable by patients who need to cope with what is happening to their own bodies and minds. This fundamental need for informed patient involvement, although long apparent[155], has not been a focus of health policy until the last decade. The escalating costs of chronic illness, however, combined with the consumer-driven care movement, have led providers, payers and consumers alike to seek ways to facilitate informed patient involvement in care. That involvement requires external standards and tools that patients themselves learn to use, both independently and jointly with their providers. Without that patient involvement, unnecessary complexity and fragmentation occur, as multiple providers intrude on inherently personal decisions that patients are better positioned to manage for themselves.

---

153 Bartholomew, note 64 above, p. 273.

154 Institute of Medicine, *Crossing the Quality Chasm*, note 146 above, p. 27.

155 Weed L. *Medical Records, Medical Education and Patient Care* (1969), note 2 above, pp. 46, 48 ("In the last analysis, the patient with a chronic disease must in large part be his own physician … patients are the largest untapped resource in medical care today"). We return to this issue in part IX.A and Appendix B below.

This need for organization and transparency in complex cases is not limited to patients and practitioners. Three broader concerns are also at stake.

First, complex cases are an essential source of new medical knowledge. By definition, complex cases are those where established knowledge does not yield quick or certain solutions. Developing new knowledge requires examining how ultimate outcomes connect with patient characteristics and provider inputs in all their minute particulars. These connections cannot be traced when the processes of care are disorganized and poorly documented.

Second, high quality performance by providers in complex cases must be made definable and reproducible comprehensively, if costs and quality are ever to be brought under control. This principle applies to both individual and institutional providers. For institutional providers, comprehensive standards of high quality must be defined, disseminated and enforced much more effectively than now occurs. For individual practitioners, medical education and credentialing must be transformed into processes that instill and enforce high standards of performance.

Third, the functioning of the health care marketplace depends on detailed standards of care defining high quality performance in complex cases. Effective price competition, for example, cannot occur when quality is variable and uncertain, because cost-quality trade-offs cannot be safely made. Disconnected from quality, mere price competition is corrosive and demoralizing, not productive and creative.

In short, complex cases present a host of difficulties and demands that may seem intractable. Yet, complex cases can in fact be managed effectively. The key is to use the medical record to organize the myriad processes of care around defined patient needs.

B. The role of the medical record in bringing order and transparency to complex cases

Recall from Part I the concept that patient care must be oriented towards a single purpose: individualized medical problem solving for unique patients. Achieving this purpose in complex cases requires, first of all, an organizing principle. Order must emerge by applying that principle to the flood of patient data over time. Accumulating data must be logically organized for rapid comprehension, and the organizing principle must be apparent to all.

The tool for organizing patient data is the medical record. Properly designed, the medical record (electronic or otherwise) makes it possible to manage and comprehend patient data in complex cases. The organizing principle is simply to follow with rigor the basic steps of orderly problem solving in any field:

(1)   gathering relevant information,

(2)   identifying and defining problems based on the initial information,

(3)   developing a plan of action for each problem in light of the other problems, and

(4)   following through on the plans, which includes gathering feedback and making adjustments as needed over time.

These steps can be viewed as the four phases of all medical action. The corresponding components of the medical record are:

(1)   a defined database,

(2)   a problem list,

(3)   plans for each problem, and

(4)   progress notes on each problem.

These four steps form a superstructure. Each step has an internal structure of components reflecting the logic of each activity. Part VI.C below explains these components in some detail.

The medical record structure based on these problem-solving steps is known as the problem-oriented medical record ("POMR"). The term "problem-oriented" has two interrelated meanings:

- the information in the medical record is organized by the patient problem to which the information relates (as distinguished from the traditional arrangement by source, with doctors' notes in one place, nurses' notes in another, lab data in another, etc.), and

- problems are defined in terms of the patient's complete medical needs rather than providers' beliefs or specialty orientation (thus, for example, the record should cover not just the "chief complaint" but all identified medical needs, and those needs should be defined in terms of the problems requiring solution, not in terms of providers' diagnostic hypotheses or treatment plans).

A source-oriented structure does little to bring order to the processes of care. It does not correspond to patient needs, nor does it reveal the context and basis and logic of provider actions, nor does it facilitate coordinated action among multiple practitioners over time, nor does it enable informed patient involvement. In contrast, a problem-oriented structure requires that all practitioners record each plan and progress note by the specific patient problem to which is relates. The patient's total medical situation is summarized by a complete problem list appearing at the first page or screen of the record. The problem list facilitates organized analysis of each problem in light of the patient's other problems, and definition of problems in terms of patient needs makes practitioners and the patient more accountable for action and inaction bearing on the whole patient's condition, including psychosocial problems. In short, the POMR standard of care governs not only the medical record but the ongoing processes of care.[156]

The POMR standard establishes an architecture, an explicit structure for organized action jointly by the patient and practitioners over time. As the Institute of Medicine has observed, the POMR standard "reflects an orderly process of problem solving, a heuristic that aids in identifying, managing and resolving patients' problems."[157] Enforcing the POMR standard means that individually relevant information is collected, considered and acted upon by all practitioners and the patient over time, with the patient's total situation taken into account every step of the way. A key element in this process is the source of informational inputs. The process becomes enormously more powerful and reliable when informational inputs are brought under control with use of knowledge coupling tools.[158]

---

156 See Stratmann, W. Assessing the Problem-Oriented Approach to Care Delivery. Medical Care. XVIII(4):456-464 (April 1980) ("the concept of comprehensive care" is "the philosophical foundation for the problem-oriented approach to care delivery. It is important to distinguish between the problem-oriented record and the problem-oriented approach to care delivery. The former is a tool; the latter, a comprehensive set of clinical and administrative guidelines.")

157 Dick R, Steen E., Detmer D. *The Computer-Based Patient Record: An Essential Technology for Health Care.* (Washington: National Academy Press, rev. 1997), pp. 90-91. These two pages are available in full text beginning at http://books.nap.edu/openbook.php?record_id=5306&page=90. Compare Robert Wachter's description of the traditional source-oriented standard (still in common use):

take a look at today's medical record, and ask yourself whether – if we could start fresh – *this* is the tool you would have constructed if your goal were to allow a diverse group of providers to collaborate while caring for terribly sick patients. In particular, would you have members of each tribe – docs, nurses, physical therapists, nutritionists – writing notes in their own style, using various totems and ritualistic phrasings, in files separated by colored dividers that might as well be electrified fences?

Of course not. In fact, today's medical record virtually guarantees the silo-ization of care. Few physicians ever read nurses' notes, even though all of us depend on the nurses to be our eyes and ears. And the situation iteratively worsens every day. Why would a nurse, realizing that no doctor ever reads her notes, even *try* to write them to be useful to physicians? And visa versa, obviously. Over the years, this divergence has been codified into ritual, calcified by templates, and hard wired through regulations whose original rationale no one can remember.

http://thehealthcareblog.com/blog/2008/01/11/creating-a-facebook-like-medical-record/

158 Some readers may be interested in the origins of the POMR and knowledge coupling software. In general terms, the POMR grew out of LLW's contrasting experiences as a clinician and as a research scientist in biochemistry. The lack of scientific rigor in clinical practice led LLW in the 1950's to begin development of the POMR. For further description, see the works cited in note 2 and the interview with LLW in the Summer 2009 issue of *The Permanente Journal* (Vol.

Examining current patient care and medical records in this light exposes an embarrassing gap between what caring for patients requires and what actual practice reveals, but it also leads to a vision for closing that gap:

1. Data collection

Required: <u>A comprehensive, defined database.</u> The database must be *comprehensive* enough not only to gather information about the "chief complaint" but also to identify other medical problems and detect incipient problems before harm occurs. The questions in the database must be explicitly *defined* in advance of the patient encounter for two reasons. First, the patient and practitioner need to know what data to collect without resort to their own judgments. Second, they need an explicit basis for the problem list (the positive and negative findings taken into account). For these standards of care to be met, ongoing quality control is required.

Revealed: Data collection is usually neither comprehensive nor defined. Even when provider institutions define a comprehensive database, reliable collection and recording of data may not be enforced in practice. Moreover, quality control may be lacking even when data are collected. The choice of data to collect may be biased by financial interests or may otherwise not reflect the best current thinking on screening and investigation, and personnel who perform physical examinations may or may not do so correctly. In recording data, practitioners often record positive

---

13, No. 3), available at http://xnet.kp.org/permanentejournal/sum09/Lawrence_Weed.html. That led to a federally funded effort in the 1960s and 1970's to develop a minicomputer-based electronic version of the POMR known as the PROMIS system. See Schultz J., A History of the PROMIS Technology: An Effective Human Interface, from Goldberg A., ed. *A History of Personal Workstations* (Reading, MA: Addison-Welsey Pub. Co. 1988), available at http://en.wikipedia.org/wiki/Problem-Oriented_Medical_Information_System. See also Weed LL., Hertzberg R. The use and construction of problem-knowledge couplers, the knowledge-coupler editor, knowledge networks and the problem-oriented medical record for the microcomputer. *IEEE Proceedings of the Seventh Annual Symposium on Computer Applications in Health Care*, 831-836. New York, IEEE Computer Society. The PROMIS system was designed to include extensive medical knowledge content, in order to overcome the mind's limited capacity for knowledge retrieval. But this information *retrieval* solution left unsolved the mind's limited capacity for information *processing*—integrating medical knowledge with patient data. This dilemma led LLW to conceive and develop knowledge coupling software as an essential complement to the POMR. LLW left the PROMIS organization and in 1982 founded Problem-Knowledge Couplers (PKC) Corporation to further develop knowledge coupling software using personal computers.

but not negative findings, making it difficult to interpret absence of a positive finding (was it negative or was it never checked?). The resulting variability in data and documentation completely undermines the next step—problem definition.

Envisioned: Knowledge coupling software would objectively and explicitly define a comprehensive database (history, physical examination and basic laboratory tests) for health risk assessment and wellness promotion. The patient history would take the form of a detailed electronic questionnaire with explanatory text and graphics so that the patient and family members could complete it on their own, taking as much time as necessary to be accurate, without consuming the time of expensive practitioners. The physical examination would be conducted by practitioners who are carefully trained and periodically audited on their skillful and reliable performance of each element of the examination. The content of the physical examination and laboratory testing, objectively determined by the knowledge coupling software, would be limited to items that are simple, quick, inexpensive and minimally invasive. The software's output would automatically be imported into electronic medical records following the POMR standard. The patient and a practitioner would jointly discuss the database entries to confirm their correctness and assess their implications, taking into account any concerns identified by the patient, family or practitioners beyond the information elicited by the software.[159]

2. Problem definition

Required: <u>A complete problem list that accounts for all abnormalities in the database.</u> Not only the chief complaint but other medical problems must be identified with completeness and defined with precision. Completeness is important for the obvious reason that unidentified medical problems may cause harm, and for the less obvious reason that diagnosis and treatment of any one problem requires considering the other medical problems and coordinating the associated medical interventions. Precision in

---

159 What is envisioned here and in the following paragraphs has been actually put into practice by Dr. Ken Bartholomew, as described in his chapter, "The Perspective of a Practitioner," in *Knowledge Coupling*, note 2 above.

defining problems is necessary to develop rational, cost-effective plans for each problem.

Revealed: A complete problem list is not achieved in most environments. This often is due to an incomplete database. But it may also be due to failure to account for all data collected and failure to consider psychosocial problems. Significant abnormalities may simply be ignored, or related data may not be synthesized into a diagnosis because the unaided mind does not recognize the relationship. The specialty training, parochial experiences and financial interests of providers may unjustifiably bias what synthesis there is. Failure to distinguish between a diagnostic hypothesis and a confirmed diagnosis may cause alternative hypotheses to be overlooked. Furthermore, since practitioners and the patient are not working together from a single, complete problem list over time, their activities are not coordinated and cumulative. All of these failings undermine rational planning for each problem.

Envisioned: Knowledge coupling software would objectively reveal the medical significance of abnormalities in the database, and thereby facilitate synthesis of related abnormalities into a diagnosis, taking all medical specialties into account. Problem lists would be subject to audit in relation to the database, creating accountability for incomplete or imprecise identification of problems. Complete, precisely defined problem lists would provide an overview of the patient's total medical condition, while serving as an index to the detailed medical record. The patient and multiple practitioners would thereby have a unified view of the patient's evolving condition over time, facilitating coordinated care.

3. Plan formulation for each problem

Required: <u>Problem-oriented plans.</u> Once the problem list is developed, each action taken should be determined as part of a written plan of action for each problem (even if the plan for some problems is to do nothing). Each plan should be labeled by the problem to which it relates and should state its rationale, in order to provide a basis for feedback. Each plan should systematically take into account the other problems on the list, the medical interventions for each, the patient's needs and goals, the best available options for addressing the problem, and the pros and cons of the various options based on the patient's individual characteristics.

Revealed: Physicians often fail to address significant patient problems even after they have been identified. In formulating plans of action for whatever problems they do address, physicians are unable to integrate all the relevant data on the patient and all the relevant diagnostic and management options from the literature, to come up with the best course of action for a unique individual. Physicians often fail to record, or even to formulate, a clear rationale for each action in relation to a specific problem, the goals to achieve, and the parameters to monitor progress towards those goals. These failures of planning and documentation completely undermine feedback. Moreover, in formulating plans, physicians do not systematically take into account problem interrelationships, the actions of other practitioners, or the patient's needs and goals.

Envisioned: Knowledge coupling software would facilitate identification of all relevant diagnostic and management options for all of the patient's problems, using patient data to determine the pros and cons of each option for that patient. The structure of the medical record would make explicit each required element of careful planning. The record would thereby expose, to the patient and the practitioners' colleagues, failure to formulate logical and complete plans directed at achieving the patient's personal goals for each problem. Informed involvement by the patient, and coordination action by practitioners, would be facilitated.

4. Follow-up on each problem

Required: Problem-oriented progress notes and flowsheets. Each plan for each problem should be carefully monitored and adjusted in light of the patient's total needs. This can only be accomplished with structured progress notes labeled by the problem to which they relate. Progress notes should be structured to enable rapid comprehension of changing data over time. For quantitative data, the required structure is usually a flowsheet. For data recorded in narrative form, the required structure should distinguish between subjective data, objective data, the practitioner's assessment, and the plan.

Revealed: Plans frequently are not well implemented , not carefully monitored and not modified based on new data. These failings occur either because required actions are not even attempted or because inadequate recording of progress notes frustrates the attempts. Without well-structured progress notes, clinicians can easily fail to recognize trends and correlations in data, lose track of significant test results, fail to consider interactions among multiple problems or fail to coordinate their activities with other practitioners. These failings occur particularly with chronic illness.

Envisioned: All practitioners would jointly maintain structured progress notes on each problem. Separately notating the course of each problem over time promotes thorough observation, feedback, follow-through and coordinated action by multiple practitioners. The structure of each note would distinguish different types of data, which tends to reveal analytical gaps and discrepancies. Numerical data and graded narrative data such as headache severity, pain severity, numbness and the like would be organized into flowsheets, thereby facilitating quick comprehension of changing parameters. Patients could better follow the course of their problems and monitor the actions of providers.

These four problem-solving steps form the basis for the POMR standard of data organization in the medical record. Part VI.C below covers the basic principles and implications of each of the above four phases of medical action and the corresponding components of the POMR.

It should not be surprising to find that recordkeeping standards of this kind have so much importance. Analogous standards of data organization in other complex activities operate as standards of thought and conduct. Publication formats for clinical trials for example, commonly require stating a pre-defined hypothesis to be tested and accurately recording the subsequent results of that testing. The same is true of the POMR (see part VI.C below). Another example is business financial records. These must conform to rigorous financial accounting standards, such as distinguishing between operating expenses and capital investment or determining when revenue can be recognized on the income statement. In the worlds of science and commerce, violating these standards has serious consequences. But medicine fails to enforce comparable standards for medical records.

"Detailed and consistent reporting has never been a strong suit of medical practitioners. Since antiquity the medical case history was more a prosaic diary for the individual physician than a scientific document meant for general readership," as Dr. Kevin Leslie has observed.[160] The Institute of Medicine has recognized that this state of affairs is unacceptable, especially with electronic medical records:

> patient records should guide and reflect clinical problem solving … the mere translation of current record formats, data and habits from paper to computer-based systems will not alone produce the range of improvements in care potentially achievable in a truly reformed patient record system. Current systems include behaviors and record forms that produce substantial waste, imprecision, and complexity in a care system less and less able to tolerate that burden. … the shift from a paper to a computer-based system offers an opportunity to study and improve clinical approaches and methods that are reflected in the record.[161]

From this perspective, the Institute of Medicine viewed the POMR standard as reflecting "an orderly process of problem-solving, a heuristic that aids in identifying, managing and resolving patients' problems." The Institute of Medicine also found "certain components of the POMR to be highly desirable in any computer-based record system. Those components include (1) a structured, systematically collected database; (2) an easily reviewed and updated problem list; and (3) routine recording of clinical formulations and plans for care and follow-up."

To reiterate, the POMR, like knowledge coupling software, is designed for individualized medical problem solving. To be reproducible and improvable, problem solving should not be *ad hoc*; rather, it should be organized, structured and explicit. In contrast to some fields (e.g. manufacturing), the output of medical problem solving must be individualized—which heightens complexity and therefore the need for order and explicit structure. When this is achieved, solutions to many of the current failings in patient care fall into place. For example, enforcing the POMR standard addresses the root causes of avoidable

160 Leslie K., Rosal J. "Standardization of the Surgical Pathology Report: Formats, Templates and Synoptic Reports." *Seminars in Diagnostic Pathology.* 11:4: 253-257 (1994).

161 Institute of Medicine, *The Computer-Based Patient Record: An Essential Technology for Health Care*, note 157 above, p. 90.

hospital readmissions.[162] More broadly, enforcing the POMR standard addresses these central failings in patient care:

- The health care system is driven by illness, not wellness, i.e., providers and patients too often neglect medical problems until they have become serious and difficult to resolve, with insufficient attention given to health maintenance (preventive care, early detection of medical problems, personal behaviors).

- Care is fragmentary and uncoordinated on two levels; first, practitioners too often fail to take into account the whole patient (all medical problems, the patient's life situation and personal goals); second, multiple practitioners too often do not communicate with each other or the patient effectively..

- Care is not patient-centered or consumer-driven; rather it is vendor-driven, with decision making in the hands of physician vendors, who are manipulated by drug and medical device vendors and third party payers.

The following discussion should be read with these issues in mind. For example, the lack of emphasis on wellness can be analyzed in terms of the first two phases of medical action—failure to maintain a defined, comprehensive database (which should always assess wellness and health habits), and failure to define a complete problem list (which should always include health maintenance as a problem). Similarly, fragmented, uncoordinated care, and care that is driven by vendor marketing rather than patient needs, can be conceived in large part as a failure to carry out the second through fourth phases of action in a problem-oriented manner.

Before turning to the details of the POMR standard, we briefly examine the current marketplace in electronic health records (EHRs). Readers familiar with that market may believe at first glance that the POMR standard is well accepted.

---

162 High rates of hospital admission within 30 days of an initial admission are widely viewed to be an indicator of poor quality and waste, but the significance of this indicator is debated. See High Readmission Rates May Not Mean Worse Hospital Care, *MedlinePlus*, July 14, 2009, at http://www.nlm.nih.gov/medlineplus/news/fullstory_101065.html (analysis showing that that a higher occurrence of readmissions after initial hospitalization for heart failure was associated with a lower, risk-adjusted 30-day death rate). In reality, the fact of avoidable readmissions and the use of such a crude indicator of quality and economy are *both* symptomatic of disorder in patient care. For further discussion of the POMR standard in relation to factors that contribute to avoidable readmissions, see Chapter 6 ("The Discharge Summary and Data Reduction") in *Knowledge Coupling*, and Chapter 7 ("The Discharge Summary") *Medical Records, Medical Education and Patient Care*, both in note 2 above.

Most EHR systems enable problem lists, and many systems allow for progress notes to be organized in the "SOAP" format prescribed by the POMR standard (see part VI.C.4). Similarly, the meaningful use standards require a problem list capability. But the POMR standard requires far more.

Failure to enforce the POMR standard has resulted in EHR products that fail to serve the most important needs of patients, practitioners and clinical researchers. The poor quality of EHR products becomes apparent when one examines their functionality for coordinating care (see our discussion of this core purpose of medical records at note 154 above). That issue was the subject of a hearing by the Meaningful Use Workgroup of the Health IT Policy Committee held August 5, 2010.[163] The hearing witnesses primarily discussed commercial EHR products marketed to physician group practices in the U.S., as distinguished from systems built in-house by some academic medical centers.

The hearing testimony pointed to one conclusion: current EHRs are falling far short of their potential to facilitate care coordination. As one practitioner testified, after enumerating the ways in which IT systems are needed to help coordinate care: "Unfortunately, even the best of the current off the shelf systems available to small practices ... do an awful job of supporting any of these."[164] Another practitioner observed: "Usability is the Achilles heel of electronic health records. ... We cannot just assume that if a piece of information is somewhere with the EHR that it will be easily accessible to the nurses and physicians caring for the patient. It may be buried in an inaccessible location or overlooked because of poor information display."[165]

---

163 The HIT Policy Committee was established under the HITECH Act provisions of the 2009 economic stimulus legislation (see note 27 above) to advise the Department of Health and Human Services (HHS). The Committee's Meaningful Use Workgroup is advising HHS on standards for EHR meaningful use, which eligible professionals and hospitals must satisfy to receive federal subsidies for EHR purchases. The written testimony cited below, along with a transcript, and audio and Webcast files are available at http://healthit.hhs.gov/portal/server.pt?open=512 &objID=1472&&PageID=17094&mode=2&in_hi_userid=11673&cached=true.

164 Testimony of Rushika Fernandopulle.

165 Testimony of Christine A. Sinsky, p. 3. She concluded with a thoughtful summary of how EHRs should contribute to coordinated care (p. 6, emphasis added):

Continuity, access and connectedness between the patient, physician and staff are the foundations of care coordination. We need *information tools that help with the broad and deep synthesis* inherent in coordinated care. We need *tools that allow the physician to see at a glance the important aspects of the patient's medical history,* be reminded of the *patient's unique psychosocial situation,* and inform decision making with *point-of-care reference knowledge.* And we need to be able to *communicate these important pieces* of the puzzle to others involved in the patient's care.

Part VI.C below describes how this vision can become reality by enforcing the POMR and

A recent article diagnosed this state of affairs as follows: "Current EMR design is heavily driven by billing and documentation needs, rather than by patient and provider needs around clinical management." Documentation needs are oriented towards legal compliance (reimbursement and litigation concerns), not quality and coordination of care. As a result, "current EMRs do little to facilitate collaborative decision making among different clinicians caring for the same patient."[166]

The question thus arises—what would EHRs look like if their design were driven by quality and coordination of care? The POMR standard, although not mentioned at the Meaningful Use Workgroup hearing, answers this question in large part. For example, the recent article on the subject mentions two specific design features of EHRs as being valuable for care coordination:

- "The problem list ... was identified by clinicians as particularly important to coordination";

- "Electronic links between the problem list and other parts of the chart containing the related care plan and notes were particularly helpful, *although this capability was uncommon.*"[167]

Both features are core elements of the POMR standard. The problem list is integrally related to another core element of the POMR—the initial database. The implications of these elements for EHRs in primary care were noted 26 years ago:

---

combinatorial standards of care and the corresponding tools.

166 O'Malley A. et al., "Are Electronic Medical Records Helpful for Care Coordination? Experiences of Physician Practices," *Journal of General Internal Medicine*, 25(3):177-185 (2010), at p. 182, 183, available at http://www.hschange.org/CONTENT/1104/OMalley.pdf. The lead author summarized this article at the Aug. 5, 2010 hearing (see the testimony of Ann O'Malley at the Web site referenced in note 163 above). Another witness similarly diagnosed the failings of current EHRs: "even the best provider facing EHRs are constructed to support the existing paradigm of care and care documentation—which is almost entirely visit and encounter based, and which ends in a legal document typically produced and attested to by a sole provider." Testimony of Peter Basch, p. 3. (These characteristics of EHRs reflect the failings of paper records. See part II.B.2.c at notes 29-30 above.) Dr. Basch further observes that "The ... Meaningful Use objectives for care coordination restrict themselves to the enablement of health information availability and mobility. [The] ... metrics are silent as to the process of care coordination ... . " In contrast, the POMR standard enables many elements of care coordination and provides a framework for enabling other elements.

167 O'Malley A. et al., cited in the preceding note, p. 179 (emphasis added). Although most EHR systems include problem lists, implementation of this feature may fall far short of the POMR standard, as discussed in part VI.C.2 below.

... since the database and problem list components of the POR [problem-oriented record] have been shown to be easily automated, a microcomputer-compatible data base and problem list might comprise important components of the primary care record suitable for the World Health Organization goal of primary care for all by the year 2000.[168]

The following discussion of the POMR reflects years of actual experience in primary care with a microcomputer-based POMR system developed by PKC Corporation and prior experience with a mini-computer-based POMR system on a hospital ward in the 1970s (as to the latter, see note 158 above). Dr. Ken Bartholomew has described his experience practicing with the PKC system as the only physician in the county in rural South Dakota (see note 2 above). Dr. Bartholomew's detailed operational description of his experience, which integrated knowledge coupling software with the electronic POMR, is highly relevant to current development of EHR meaningful use standards.

C. The medical record and the four phases of medical action

1. The database

The need for a defined, comprehensive database arises in two contexts, as discussed in Part IV.A: (1) *screening* to identify medical problems, and (2) *initial workup* of problems identified by the screening or by the patient. In both contexts, medical knowledge is coupled with patient data. This knowledge coupling function, whether carried out by the unaided mind, software tools or both, generates a database for decision making.[169]

As discussed in Part IV, the quality of decision making for an identified medical problem depends on the database created by the initial workup of that problem. Equally important is the screening database. A sound screening database should enable the patient and all practitioners to have a comprehensive view of health status. More specifically:

- The screening database should elicit enough data to discover all medical problems, not just data relevant to the "chief complaint" (see the discussion of a complete problem list in the next section).

---

168 Margolis C. et al., Increase in Relevant Data after Introduction of a Problem-Oriented Record System in Primary Pediatric Care. *Amer. J. Pub. Health*, 74(12):1410-1412 (Dec. 1984). Fifteen years before that article, the first book on the POMR discussed computerization at length (see note 2 above).

169 This section draws on *Knowledge Coupling*, note 2 above, pp. 23-80.

- The data collected should be enough to detect existing problems at an early stage, but not necessarily enough information to solve or manage each problem.

- The data collected should enable wellness assessment, that is, identification of risk factors, behaviors and living circumstances that indicate possible future health problems.

- The data collected should include not just medical data but other data about the patient's social and economic circumstances that may bear on medical decisions.

A screening database designed to achieve these purposes has two basic components: a patient profile and a review of body systems. Specifically:

- The patient profile briefly describes the patient's family situation, living circumstances, employment and financial status, and how he or she spends a routine day. These data are essential for the practitioner to understand the patient's ability to cope with medical problems and to work realistically with the patient in setting goals and planning for diagnosis and management.

- The review of body systems includes a personal and family medical history, a physical examination and laboratory tests. A well-designed review of body systems is highly cost-effective, because each finding, when abnormal, is a possible clue to at least one and usually numerous possible medical problems, including problems for which early detection would avoid serious harm and expensive care. A finding of high blood pressure, for example, suggests scores of significant possible diagnoses to investigate.

After the screening database is completed, initial workups are performed for abnormal findings as to which detailed investigation appears advisable.

To summarize, a complete initial database includes a screening database plus a set of initial workups that encompass the chief complaint, other abnormalities uncovered in the screening database and any other medical problems identified by the patient.

Like an initial workup, the screening database involves three steps (see part IV.B), each of which should be guided by knowledge coupling software:

1. Choosing initial data for assessing health status;

2. Collecting the chosen data (doing the patient/family history, physical examination and laboratory tests);

3. Identifying implications of the data.

The following brief description of PKC Corporation's Coupler for Health History Screening shows the scope of a comprehensive, defined screening database. The Coupler covers 774 findings, elicited by questions grouped in the following categories:

Body Systems Review: Present and Past Health Problems
Mental Health and Emotional Well Being
Personal Self-Care, Immunizations, Allergies
Medical Care Providers, Medications, Surgery, Imaging
Environmental Exposures, Family Disease History

The Coupler also gives the patient ample opportunity to enter information about problems and concerns not addressed in the questionnaire. The Coupler output is presented as a list of management strategies or options, listed under one or more of the following headings:

Guidance You Can Follow on Your Own
Guidance to Discuss With Your Healthcare Provider
Screenings and Tests to Discuss With Your Healthcare Provider (a list of routine
    screening tests and, if indicated, selected diagnostic tests)
Immunizations Due
Organization of Patient's Responses Into Management Categories

Evaluate Now	(a list of symptoms, problems, or concerns that should be investigated now or should receive timely follow-up)
Observe Over Time	(a list of problems or diagnoses that may require periodic re-evaluation regarding disease progression, recurrence, or management)

Monitor Risk Factors	(a list of health characteristics that may increase one's risk of having or developing a disease. Risk factors include health behaviors (for example, smoking), family health history, environmental exposures, certain past diseases (for example, polio), and severe allergic reactions (for example, bee sting).
Other Couplers to Run	(a list of diagnostic and management Couplers that will provide additional guidance on current problems and known conditions)

Suggestions to the Provider for Follow-Up (patient-reported physical findings that should be confirmed and evaluated during the physical examination)

Drugs Currently Being Taken (a list of drugs including prescription, over-the-counter, and alternative or herbal remedies)

Allergies	(a list of known allergies and allergic reactions)

Current Healthcare Providers

Current Alternative Health Providers

Documentation to Obtain for the Medical Record

Each positive response to questionnaire items is coupled to one or more of the guidance options in the foregoing categories, so that a finding is presented as a reason to implement a particular guidance option. The output of this coupling process shows information for future monitoring (e.g., exposure to workplace toxins) and further action to pursue (e.g. use of the hypertension Coupler). The output not only identifies medical problems to be investigated but also provides a wellness guide for the patient to act on, individualized to the patient's specific needs. This Coupler output should be reviewed together by the patient and practitioner, and the patient should retain a copy for later reference. In addition, the Coupler output should be used to begin or expand a personal medical record to help structure regular medical checkups.[170]

What has just been described is far different from current practice. For most patients, different providers collect a different database, each being incomplete

---

170 PKC also provides a Periodic Health Evaluation Screening Coupler to be used periodically after initial use of the Health History Screening Coupler. In addition, PKC provides the following specialized screening Couplers: Adolescent Wellness Visit (11-18 years), Adolescent Wellness (Parent's Questionnaire), International Travel Health, Lab Test Result Interpretation, Mental Health Screening, and Musculoskeletal Screening (Strength, Flexibility, Posture). See www.pkc.com.

in infinitely variable ways. The provider's concerns (or those of a third party payer) rather than the patient's needs may determine the scope of the database. Some specialists may limit themselves to working up problems within their specialty. Some may not concern themselves with a screening database, and their initial workups may overlook data needed to assess the patient's interacting problems and treatments from other medical specialties. Primary care physicians may provide episodic care focusing on whatever "chief complaint" the patient raises. They may recommend that the patient get a "complete physical," but patients often ignore the advice. When patients act on the advice, the screening database their physician collects may be perfunctory. Not all body systems may be thoroughly covered, emotional problems may not be addressed, and relevant personal characteristics and circumstances (e.g., literacy, financial difficulties, family conflicts, job stresses, health threats in the workplace and local environment) may not be taken into account.

When hospitalization occurs, the database collection process often starts anew, with little regard to data already collected elsewhere. The multiplicity of personnel in hospitals escalates disarray in database collection. This failing is especially severe in teaching hospitals. As Dr. Willis Hurst has described it:

> In a medical school environment it is not uncommon for a medical student, intern, resident, fellow and senior staff member all to be assigned to a hospitalized patient. In the past it was customary for each of these individuals to "write up" a separate account of their examination. Little time was spent by the senior staff members in determining whether there was agreement or disagreement between observers. Should a patient be readmitted to the hospital a week later, the ritual was repeated. There could be as many as six "histories" and "physicals" on the chart. There was little effort spent in judging if the database was complete and accurate. Such was not possible even when the effort was spent, since there had been no prior agreement reached regarding a defined database.[171]

Disarray in database collection is equally great outside the hospital. Medical data are collected for caregiving purposes by solo practitioners, large group practices, HMOs, dental and vision care providers, in-house medical clinics at large employers, "convenience" or "urgent care" clinics, school and university health clinics, community health centers, osteopaths, chiropractors, independent nurse practitioners, alternative medicine practitioners and others. Much data

---

171 Hurst, JW. "How Does One Develop a Defined Data Base? Who Collects the Data?", chapter 6 in *The Problem-Oriented System*, J. Willis Hurst and H. Kenneth Walker, eds. New York: Medcom Press, 1972.

collection takes place for worker's compensation and other occupational health programs that are not integrated with employer group health coverage. Other data collection occurs for purposes of employee benefit programs that often accompany basic group health coverage, including disease and disability management, employee assistance programs and wellness promotion.

To overcome this disarray, all data collection must feed into a single, integrated, electronic medical record for each person.[172] The foundation for each person's record must be a defined, comprehensive database maintained over time. Without that foundation, relevant data will not be accessible when needed, or will be duplicated unnecessarily. Most important, without the foundation of a unitary database for the whole person, patient care cannot become truly "patient-centered" or "consumer-driven." Care will always be provider-driven (or payer driven) as long as decisions are made (or imposed) based on superficial data collection serving the immediate interests of providers and payers rather than patients' total needs. To protect against that outcome, the POMR standard for initial data collection *identifies* the patient's total needs, and thereby makes accountability possible.[173]

To reiterate, the unitary database must be comprehensive and it must be defined. Both requirements are worth discussing further.

"Comprehensive" does not mean exhaustive. "Comprehensive" means that the initial database should cover every body system, plus external circumstances relevant to medical decision making, plus diagnostic or treatment options worth considering for identified problems. This comprehensiveness is necessary to escape the tunnel vision otherwise fostered by provider specialization (as discussed further below). Comprehensiveness does not require costly or invasive procedures at the outset of care. On the contrary, the initial database should include only readily available and productive data. Productive data are data

---

172 "[T]o really improve transitions in care, what we need is a single source of truth, that is, one medical record, accessible to providers with permission, and owned by the patient. Otherwise, we perpetuate electronically what we currently have on paper: multiple medical records, each one providing only part of the story. ... In some countries in the developing world, patients bring their chart to every office visit. ... [This] actually solves several problems we have yet to solve: there is one source of truth, there is health information exchange, and it is clear that patients own and are responsible for their medical information." Testimony of Jeffrey L. Schnipper at the Meaningful Use Workgroup hearing reference in note 163 above.

173 See Margolis C. et al., Increase in Relevant Data after Introduction of a Problem-Oriented Record System in Primary Pediatric Care, note 168 above ("our findings show that when the standardized data base and problem list components of the POR are introduced as part of a complete POR system that also includes problem-oriented progress notes and regular audit, both data collection and chronic problem identification in a community clinic are significantly improved").

that, when coupled with medical knowledge, generate the maximum amount of useful information at the least possible risk, discomfort and cost.

"Defined" means that the data to be collected must be spelled out in advance and then accurately recorded. Unless its scope is thus defined, and unless actual data collection (or lack of collection) is recorded, then the basis for subsequent decision making is uncertain, and quality control is undermined. This does not mean that all defined data must be collected uniformly without regard to time and resource constraints. Rather, it means that any omissions should be deliberately considered and then documented, so that the subsequent decision making can take the information gap into account. This documentation should be an automatic byproduct of the tools used to generate the database, and the tool should preserve all questions presented and the user's responses.

Not only practitioners but patients and third party payers need to apply these principles. Patients sometimes ignore advice to get a thorough screening database or initial workup, and third party payers typically do not pay for the time investment required from providers. This short-term thinking is counterproductive in both medical and economic terms. Even from a short-term perspective, a thorough database becomes relatively affordable if non-physician personnel do most of the data collection (yet, both regulatory and reimbursement systems inhibit this efficiency). Moreover, from a long term perspective, the up-front investment of time in collecting a carefully designed, thorough database may well pay for itself if its results are acted upon intelligently.

Human nature, of course, often leads us to act in the short term and neglect the long term. Some people, for example, go for many years without ever seeing a primary care provider to obtain a screening database, simply due to neglect and inertia. The solution is to create short-term incentives to change such behavior. This solution is increasingly recognized by employers and other third party payers that adopt wellness programs with financial incentives. But they must do more than create incentives for behavior change. They must also bring about reforms assuring that a thorough initial database is provided to consumers who seek it, and is part of the standard of care that providers are expected to follow.

Privacy concerns or personal sensitivities sometimes make patients unwilling to disclose or discuss sensitive information called for by a complete screening database or initial workup. To some extent, knowledge coupling software accommodates this concern, because questions can be answered with "uncertain" as well as "yes" or "no." This leaves ambiguous the patient's condition on the point in question, and allows for the possibility that enough other detailed data will be collected to resolve the question without disclosure of the sensitive point. In some circumstances, however, an unavoidable trade-off exists between privacy and disclosing accurate data. This reality highlights the need for effective privacy protections to minimize the tradeoffs. To the extent a trade-off is unavoidable, patients must make a choice. But the present system leaves patients with a Hobson's choice between, on the one hand, withholding accurate data and compromising medical decision making, or, on the other, disclosing accurate data with no assurance that the data are truly needed or likely to be used intelligently. If patients have that assurance and if they are informed of the precise relevance of the data at issue, then they can rationally decide whether the benefits of accurate data collection outweigh personal privacy concerns.

2. The problem list

At the heart of medical decision making in complex cases should be construction of a problem list.[174] Its most basic function is simply to serve as a table of contents to the record. The utility of problem lists was so obvious that they became a common practice soon after the concept was introduced. But problem lists are usually not carefully defined or complete, due to lack of standards and enforcement for medical recordkeeping. Problem lists are treated as a convenience, not a discipline.[175]

Problem lists must satisfy two distinct requirements—analytical precision and thoroughness. First, each problem on the list must be defined at a level the current data support. Second, the problem list must be complete; that is, it must account for all abnormalities in the initial database as well as problems otherwise identified by the patient and practitioner. Failure to satisfy both requirements undermines order and transparency in complex cases.

---

174 This section draws on *Knowledge Coupling*, note 2 above, pp. 81-99. For further discussion, see *The Problem-Oriented System*, note 171, and its successor volume, *Applying the Problem-Oriented System* (1973).

175 Even the convenience of serving as a table of contents to the record is lost when plans and progress notes are not linked to the problems to which they relate, as is commonly the case with commercial EHRs. See note 167 above. In contrast, making the linkage between the problem list and the body of the record not only serves the purposes discussed in this section but also facilitates segmentation of EHRs for privacy purposes. See 42 USC § 300jj.12(b)(2)(B)(i) (a new provision added to the Public Health Service Act by the HITECH Act that requires the HIT Policy Committee to make recommendations on data segmentation in EHRs for protecting sensitive information) and Benaloh, et al., Patient-Controlled Encryption: Ensuring Privacy of Electronic Medical Records (Nov. 2009, Cloud Computing Security Workshop) (need to categorize medical data so that patient can delegate access to chosen subsets of data), available at http://research.microsoft.com/pubs/102475/PCE-CCSW.pdf.

a. Defining medical problems

What does analytical precision mean in defining medical problems? As stated above, the basic concept is that problems should be defined at a level objectively justified by current data. This is a fundamental tenet of the POMR standard. Thus, a diagnostic hypothesis should not appear on the problem list unless and until data are obtained confirming the hypothesis. Until then, the problem list should include one or more abnormalities for which diagnostic hypotheses are possible explanations.[176] The diagnostic hypotheses should appear not on the problem list but as part of the physician's planning for diagnostic investigation (as discussed in part VI.C.3). Knowledge coupling software simplifies this process greatly, because it helps identify diagnostic possibilities, and what data points are sufficient to confirm any one of those possibilities.

The best available guidance from the literature is often equivocal as applied to unique individual patients. In the many cases where medical science is uncertain, confirmation of a hypothesis may not be possible; stated differently, different clinicians may reach different conclusions from the same data points. But this difficulty is not a failing of the POMR standard or knowledge coupling software. It is a reality of medicine that those tools expose. Medical uncertainty and judgmental differences among clinicians become far more manageable if those clinicians precisely distinguish between their hypotheses and their conclusions. Departures from this principle are a root cause of confusion, oversight and lack of follow-up in patient care. Placing a diagnostic possibility in the patient's problem list, and labeling it as a problem rather than as a hypothesis, channels thinking towards that one possibility. The numerous other possibilities suggested by the abnormal findings are not thoroughly considered. Abnormal findings that don't fit the diagnostic judgment tend to be left off the problem list. Then they are easily neglected as subjects for follow-up investigation. And the record fails to make any of this clear.

The vital importance of diagnostic follow-up is suggested by a recent study of missed and delayed diagnoses. Based on retrospective analysis of 307 closed malpractice claims, the study found that "failure to create a proper follow-up

---

176 This concept is absent from the final EHR "meaningful use" and certification standards regulations issued by the Office of National Coordinator (ONC) for Health IT. The preamble to the meaningful use regulations describes a problem list as "a list of current and active diagnoses as well as past diagnoses relevant to the current care of the patient." 75 Fed. Reg. 44336 (July 28, 2010). Nothing in the current "Stage 1" regulation defines standards for problem formulation.

Failure to enforce the POMR standard in current EHRs is evident from the following in Dr. O'Malley's article (note 166 above): "clinicians complained that problem lists grew 'exponentially' and became 'cluttered with redundant and irrelevant information' as EMRs automatically listed diagnostic codes related to each new test" (p. 179).

plan" was the second of "the leading breakdown points in the diagnostic process" (the first was failure to order an appropriate diagnostic test).[177] In contrast, the Institute of Medicine has written that "the chance of follow-up for a problem listed in the problem list is significantly greater" with the POMR than with non-problem-oriented record formats.[178] And the "chance of follow-up" is no longer a matter of chance when an enforceable standard of care exists for a complete problem list linked to plans and progress notes for each problem.

The traditional medical record does not clearly link initial data to the physician's plans for further action[179], nor does the record clearly show the physician's thinking about either. This approach to documenting thought and action in the medical record completely undermines order, transparency and quality control in complex cases.

Consider a patient with apparent heart failure. If the initial findings convince the physicians that no other possibilities than heart failure are worth considering, then the POMR standard would not permit the physician simply to proceed on that basis. Instead, the POMR standard would require the physician to document the conclusion reached and the reasons for it. More specifically, the physician would enter heart failure on the problem list, and would also explain in the record the findings on which this diagnosis is based.

In addition to carefully defining each problem on the problem list in a manner supported by the data (the *basis* for the problem statement), it is important also to define the *status* of the problem and the *disability* resulting from the problem. Specifying a problem's basis, status and disability can be regarded as part of defining the problem. These elements of a problem's definition, however, are not placed on the problem list. Rather they are placed in the initial plan for the problem, because each of these elements must be taken into account when formulating the plan. Accordingly, we discuss these elements in part VI.C.3 below on initial plans.

The required analysis and documentation are much more readily accomplished where knowledge coupling software is used to generate the initial database. The software displays all of the diagnostic possibilities worth considering for the patient and all of the associated findings, positive and negative, for each possibility. In a simple case, as postulated in this scenario, enough of the expected findings for heart failure would be positive, and most of the expected findings for other

---

177 Gandhi T. et al., Missed and Delayed Diagnoses in the Ambulatory Setting, note 6 above.

178 *The Computer-Based Patient Record*, note 157 above, p. 90. See Starfield et al., Coordination of care and its relation to continuity and medical records. Med Care 15:929-938 (1977).

179 This is still the case with many current EHRs; see note 167 above.

diagnostic possibilities worth considering would be negative, so that the physician could reasonably judge that heart failure has occurred. The physician would simply export this Coupler output (the diagnostic possibilities and associated findings) from the Coupler into the POMR, thereby documenting the basis of the diagnostic conclusion. This information in the POMR would be labeled by the problem to which it relates, so that any other party could immediately see its relevance and evaluate the physician's diagnostic conclusion.

It is important to understand the synergistic interrelationship among the initial database, the problem list and knowledge coupling software. Without use of knowledge coupling software to generate the initial database, the detailed initial findings needed to recognize all the diagnostic possibilities would likely not be made at the outset of care. Even if the necessary findings were made, physicians would be unlikely to evaluate them correctly because the number of findings and diagnostic possibilities to sort out is usually prohibitive for the unaided mind in complex cases. It is true that experienced physicians might correctly surmise the correct diagnosis with or without detailed data collection and use of knowledge coupling software. But their surmise would be only an educated guess. Neither the physician nor the patient nor third parties should be confident in this guess without systematically working through all potentially relevant diagnostic possibilities and the detailed patient findings relevant to assessing them. If that careful analysis is undertaken and documented, then everyone concerned can be confident in the diagnostic conclusion.

b. Scope of the problem list

In constructing a problem list the physician must not only define each problem correctly but also assure that the list is complete in relation to the initial database.[180] Without a comprehensive database, no problem list can be complete. With a comprehensive database, the problem list is complete if it accounts for all the abnormalities in the database as well as any other problems identified by the practitioner and patient.

---

180 This concept of completeness is absent from the final EHR standards and certification regulation requirements for problem lists, issued by ONC. According to the regulation's preamble, "the problem list must be comprehensive in the sense that it must be capable of including entries provided over an extended period of time. Consequently, for [EHRs] to be certified for an ambulatory setting, they will need to be designed to enable the user to electronically record, modify and retrieve a patient's problem list over multiple encounters." 75 Fed. Reg. 64604 (July 28, 2010). In the meaningful use regulation, for the objective of maintaining an up-to-date problem list," the Stage 1 compliance measure is simply that more than 80% of patients have at least one entry on the problem list. 45 CFR 495.6(d)(3)(ii), 75 Fed. Reg. 44567 (July 28, 2010). This is a remarkably rudimentary concept of a complete problem list.

The problem list can account for abnormalities in the database in either of two ways. Each abnormality can appear on the list as a problem in itself, or it can be one element of the stated basis of a problem on the list.

Omission of a problem and its serious consequences are illustrated by a case involving surgery for a bladder tumor.[181] The surgery revealed that the bladder tumor had spread to the colon. That required bringing the surgery to a halt, and resuming it later after further consideration of how to proceed. Yet, the patient should never have been exposed to this increased risk and expense. The initial database had revealed a history of bloody stools with intermittent constipation and diarrhea. Those database findings were never accounted for on the problem list. Had these findings been recorded as a problem to investigate, then the tumor's spread to the colon might have been established, or at least anticipated as a possibility, before the surgery was undertaken. The surgical team could then have determined in advance how to deal with the colon's involvement.

This case illustrates two reasons a complete problem list is essential. First, problems missing from the list will likely be neglected until they become obvious and more harmful. Second, proper analysis, planning and follow-up for each problem depends on awareness of the patient's other problems, the potential interactions and unmet needs associated with each. For example, radiologists who have worked with problem-oriented records find that the problem list greatly facilitates interpretation of clinical images.[182] The problem list is thus simultaneously reductionist and holistic, providing the benefits of both perspectives.

The discipline of a complete problem list is essential to maintain the medical record's credibility as an information tool. When a physician encounters abnormalities in patient data not accounted for in the problem list, the likely reaction is distrust of the record. This distrust tends to provoke the physician into redoing data collection and reformulating the portions of the problem list and plans. This duplication of effort and indecisiveness are not only wasteful but also create unease in patients. The larger point is that enforcing a complete problem list tends to bring accountability to the entire process of care, very much as enforcing generally accepted accounting standards in the preparation of financial statements tends to bring accountability to business operations.

Perhaps the most frequent and most serious omission from problem lists is social and psychiatric problems. These omissions are critical, not only because

---

181 This case is described in *Knowledge Coupling*, note 2 above, pp. 93-94.

182 See the text at notes 75-77 above regarding the utility of a detailed clinical history for radiologists. The problem list captures the history information that is most relevant for the radiologist's purposes.

those problems are important to address in themselves but also because they are essential to consider in diagnosing[183], and managing other problems that originate from purely organic causes. Awareness of these connections is missing among practitioners who fail to account for social and psychiatric problems in developing problem lists. This in turn compromises the growth of medical knowledge (see part VII.B below) and improvement of public health.[184]

Public health measures in the developed world over the last 150 years have radically reduced many infectious diseases. These conditions plagued disadvantaged social classes. But now, Dr. Nortin Hadler argues, the disadvantaged still bear the brunt of pathological social conditions that remain endemic. The health care system, oriented to treating personal health problems, cannot remedy the social conditions in which those problems become uncontrollable. In Dr. Hadler's words: "Health-adverse behaviors and cardiovascular risk factors may relate to the proximate cause of death, but they account for less than 25 percent of the hazard to longevity." The remaining 75 percent, Dr. Hadler argues, is attributable to "life-course hazards that powerfully perturb our biology and our fate. Much of this threat can be captured by measurements of our socioeconomic status (SES)."[185] Dr. Hadler sheds further light on the historical relationship between social disadvantage, health status and the health care system:

> The great German pathologist Rudolf Virchow (1821-1902) developed a notion of "natural" as opposed to "artificial" diseases and epidemics. He considered typhus, scurvy and tuberculosis to be "artificial" because they were primarily due to social conditions. "The artificial epidemics … strike therefore primarily those classes that do not enjoy the advantages of the culture."

> The stratum of society that dies before its time falls victim to "artificial epidemics," which account for 75 percent of mortal hazard. These epidemics will not respond to pharmaceuticals, nor can they be surgically excised. They play out well beyond the walls of the clinic and the hospital. They are not considered the proper target of the "Health Promotion – Disease Prevention" initiatives of contemporary medicine.[186]

---

183 Almost every diagnostic Coupler that PKC Corporation has developed includes social and psychiatric conditions among the diagnostic possibilities to take into account.

184 *Knowledge coupling*, note 2 above, pp. 88-90.

185 Hadler N. *The Last Well Person: How to Stay Well Despite the Health Care System* (Montreal: McGill-Queen's University Press, 2004), p. 11.

186 *Ibid.*, p. 12.

Dr. Hadler goes on to illuminate the contemporary artificial epidemics that he argues "threaten our longevity far more than such recognized causes as hypertension, obesity and or adult onset diabetes." These unrecognized epidemics are associated with low socioeconomic status and harmful conditions of employment:

> A lifetime tottering on the edge of poverty is a lifetime likely to be mean, often discouraging, sometimes desperate—and often short. What is it about a compromised socioeconomic status (SES) that is so malevolent? Multiple psychosocial factors have emerged from studies of relative poverty. Some of these factors operate from conception, but the majority derive from the loss of self-respect and the resentment, if not hostility, that results from the sense of abject vulnerability associated with and imposed by poverty. A few are associated with nutrition and life-stage maturation. Much remains unknown, but it is clear that the array of psychosocial challenges to be faced day after day in poverty, and that prove insurmountable, levy a heavier toll on health and longevity than any other factor in the 'advanced' world. Poverty in nations that are not resource-challenged is a reproach to both their political systems and their public health agendas.

> Employment itself is no generic solution to the malevolence of poverty. Some facts of life in modern workforces rival the psychosocial aspects of poverty in extracting a toll on healthfulness and longevity. A consistent story is starting to emerge, with major implications for the health of the public.[187]

The health care system cannot change basic social, economic and cultural conditions. But the health care system can help document the harmful externalities associated with those conditions. In that way, the health care system can inform political and economic choices made in the public and private sectors. Imagine a community where providers collectively maintain rigorous medical records with complete problem lists documenting precisely how health problems are associated with harmful living and employment conditions, and thus showing how reform of those local conditions would improve the health and economic status of the community. In that environment it is not hard to imagine strong public and private support for reform. In contrast, the current environment engenders resistance to reform by those who benefit from the

---

187 *Ibid.*, pp. 166-67.

status quo and those who see no hope of a return on investing the resources that would be needed to improve harmful living or employment conditions..

Equally important, the health care system can engender greater public and private support for itself by expending scarce resources with the maximum possible effectiveness, and by helping individuals cope more effectively with their own physical and psychological frailties. Now that the health reform legislation is moving us towards universal coverage, millions of people will enter the system and create greater demand for medical resources. Their neglected needs must be identified and efficiently addressed. That will never happen with the present uncontrollable, unproductive, unaffordable non-system of care.

3. Initial plans

For each problem on the problem list, an initial plan of action must be considered.[188] This point may seem too obvious to be worth making. Yet, "physicians generally have no clue about what a care plan is, why it would be needed, and why they should bother with such a thing." (In contrast, "nurses grew up with this concept of a care plan and documenting, keeping it up to date and so on as part of what they do."[189])

This point reminds us that the POMR's explicit structure, in contrast to unstructured clinical judgment, brings order and transparency to patient care. The very appearance of a problem list at the beginning of the record protects against overlooking the need to plan for each problem,[190] just as the record of a defined database protects against overlooking abnormal findings that should be accounted for in the problem list.

More fundamentally, the POMR structure promotes accountability in cases where the need for a plan is neglected. The absence of plan for a stated problem is made obvious to the providers involved, to outside parties (peer reviewers, regulators, third party payers), and, most important, to patients themselves. Here we see one of the many ways in which patients and their advocates can use the POMR standard of care to monitor and enforce quality. Patients can demand that problems not be ignored, they can participate in developing

---

188 This section draws on *Knowledge Coupling*, note 2 above, pp. 81-99.

189 Testimony of Gordon Schectman, Meaningful Use Workgroup hearing transcript, note 163 above, p. 61.

190 See Hartung D., et al. Clinical Implications of an Accurate Problem List on Heart Failure Treatment. *J Gen Intern Med.* 2005;20(2):143-147, available at www.medscape.com/view-article/502880 ("Accurate documentation of heart failure on the problem list of patients with known systolic dysfunction is associated with a significant increase in the likelihood of being prescribed medications with known clinical benefit").

initial plans, and they can thus become more informed about and personally committed to acting on those plans. That kind of patient involvement not only improves quality and patient satisfaction but also helps practitioners avoid error and malpractice litigation.

Some may object that requiring a plan for every problem will generate excessive or unnecessary care. This objection misconceives what is required. The POMR standard demands only that a plan for each problem be explicitly considered and recorded, not that action be taken. Very often the best plan is to take no action or to defer action.

An obvious example is a terminally ill patient with multiple problems. The best plan for most of those problems may be to do nothing other than palliative care to ease the patient's suffering. Another example is a deteriorating diabetic who smokes and has multiple other problems that either do not require immediate attention or cannot be successfully treated as long as the diabetes and smoking problems are out of control. The best plans for those other problems might be to do nothing until the patient successfully completes a smoking cessation program and achieves better control of her blood sugar level. A practitioner in a busy clinic could confront the patient with an explicit plan in her medical record that spending scarce time and resources on treatments for secondary problems cannot be justified as long as the patient persists with self-destructive neglect of her smoking and diabetes. Such a plan of action motivates the patient, establishes a basis for measuring progress and uses scarce resources productively.[191]

Moreover, the explicit plan promotes accountability in a broader way. Returning to the example of the diabetic smoker, suppose one of the patient's secondary problems is a minor skin condition and that the patient is unwilling or unable to pay for its treatment herself. Suppose further that the patient waits until her insurance deductible for the year is satisfied and then goes to a dermatologist. Seeing a lucrative opportunity, the dermatologist ignores the patient's medical record, undertakes an expensive treatment program, does not contact the patient's other physician, does not consider how the skin treatment program interacts with the diabetes care and submits the bill to the patient's insurer. The insurer accesses the patient's medical record, concludes that paying for the skin treatment is not justifiable in the context of patient's problem list and plans, and refers the whole matter to a peer review organization for review of the dermatologist's practice. This example illustrates how the explicit, intelligible structure of the POMR standard promotes accountability at many levels.

To reiterate, the POMR standard involves both a superstructure (the four basic components previously described) and the internal structure of each

191 For examples, see Dr. Ken Bartholomew's description, note 64 above, p. 265.

component. For the initial plans component, the first level of internal structure is that each problem identified on the problem list requires a separate plan (even if that plan is to do nothing). The next level is that each plan should include the components listed below. In the electronic version of the POMR, these components are known as an element set. The element set for initial plans is made up of the following:

```
Basis
Status
Disability
Goal
Follow course:
        Parameters to monitor course and status of problem
        Parameters to monitor response to therapy
Investigate further:
        Hypotheses to be investigated
        Measures to investigate each hypothesis
Complications to watch for
```

The POMR software calls up this element set when the user formulates initial plans, thereby disciplining the user to be organized and complete, while facilitating feedback and quality control by the patient and third parties. Knowledge coupling software can provide crucial guidance in this process—for example, by suggesting specific parameters, hypotheses or complications to consider.

A complete discussion of each of these elements is beyond the scope of this book. The following points, however, should be understood.

As noted in Part VI.C.2.a, the Basis, Status and Disability elements can be regarded as elements of each problem's definition. Because these elements must be kept in mind when formulating plans, they are placed in the Initial Plans component of the record. Note the following about each element:

- The *basis* of the problem statement is one or more abnormalities in the database that constitute evidence objectively justifying the problem statement. When the practitioner uses knowledge coupling software to generate the database, the software's output automatically states the positive findings associated with the problem, avoiding idiosyncratic variations in selection and description of associated findings.

- The *status* of the problem is a statement of whether the problem is getting worse, better or staying the same. Including this element in electronic records makes it possible at any time to generate a listing of patients and problems that are getting worse, which is useful for setting priorities and budgeting time.

- The *disability* resulting from the problem is often the primary concern of the patient and the primary focus of management efforts by ancillary practitioners such as physical therapists. Stating the disability requires the practitioner to identify the problem's significance from the patient's perspective. For example, a shoulder problem might require absence from work for a manual laborer but not for an office worker. In addition, stating the disability may affect the other elements discussed below.

The next element of planning is a goal statement. This helps ensure that the problem is cost-effectively handled in a patient-centered manner. Practitioners must always ask themselves—is what we are doing *to* the patient being done *for* the patient? Stated differently, patients must ask their providers—does what you propose for my problem make sense for me, considering my other problems, and circumstances and preferences? Particularly when specialists are involved, it is all too easy to fall into medical activity that is driven by provider habits or interests, not individual patient needs. An explicit goal statement is essential to protect patients from this tendency. In setting goals for each problem, two principles should be followed:

- *The goal should be determined in light of the complete problem list and the patient profile element of the database.* Otherwise, the medical activity that results might well be pointless or contraindicated. If, for example, the problem list includes terminal carcinoma of the lung, then the goal for a hypertension problem may not be to lower the blood pressure to normal limits.

- *The patient must be involved when goals are set.* The patient is often in the best position to set priorities and weigh trade-offs when deciding how to pursue any one problem in light of the others. Sometimes pursuing the medically ideal approach to all problems simultaneously is more than the patient can cope with. The patient needs to be informed about what is involved and then decide what he or she can handle and when. Morale is achievement and achievement depends on reasonable goals set by the patient.

The next element of planning is a statement of how to follow the course of the problem and its treatment (if any). This element is of paramount importance because it establishes feedback loops. The provider must identify parameters and set thresholds that reveal the problem's status (getting worse, better or staying the same) and alert decision makers to the need for corrective action. Carelessness in this element undermines safety, quality and cost control in a host of different ways. For example:

- Rapidly advancing problems can escalate into unnecessary emergencies or fatalities because no one watched simple parameters frequently but instead relied on a faulty diagnostic guess or elaborate test results that would be equivocal or not available until after the problem gets out of control.

- Not infrequently, physicians order tests and acquire data out of proportion to their ability to monitor, interpret and act on the results effectively. It is better to reliably monitor a few carefully chosen parameters at regular intervals than to plan a whole battery of parameters that may not be followed with care. Quality is more important than quantity.

- All too frequently, treatments are brought to a halt not by a conscious, timely, judicious decision but rather by some crisis resulting from a treatment allowed to go on too long. To avoid this, the provider needs to identify criteria for a treatment's success or failure. If such an endpoint is difficult to define, the treatment may not be worth the risk of undertaking it.

- Frequency of measurement is critical. Providers sometimes fail to consider the expected rate of change in a parameter in determining the frequency of its measurement. Or they may not recognize that when the rate of change increases, the frequency of measurement may need to increase correspondingly or a decision maker may need to be alerted.

- If more than two or three parameters and treatments need to be monitored at one time, practitioners can quickly be flooded with lab reports and other data. To handle this, practitioners need at the outset to set up flowsheets for presenting data in readily comprehensible form, as discussed in the next section.

- Parameters chosen for one problem can easily be rendered uninterpretable or invalid by the treatment or course of another problem on the list. Too much time and money are frequently spent on data that, with a little attention to interacting problems and treatments, would never have been collected.

Coping with these difficulties necessitates meticulous attention to the initial plan for setting parameters to monitor. Typically it is useful to plan in two steps for each problem: first, determine the ideal approach for the problem in isolation, and then adjust that approach based on systematic analysis of anticipated interactions with other problems and treatments. Knowledge coupling software provides detailed plan option guidance to facilitate this process.

The next element of initial planning is investigation, that is, formulating hypotheses to investigate plus the steps and sequence of investigation, in light of the goal established for the problem. If the problem is an unexplained symptom to diagnose, the plan should state diagnostic possibilities and observations or tests to investigate them. If and when the investigation generates sufficient evidence to confirm one hypothesis and rule out the others, then the problem statement should be reformulated (stating the confirmed diagnosis rather than the symptom). Similarly; the basis for the problem should be revised (stating the supporting evidence for the diagnosis rather than the symptom findings). If the problem is a condition for which the best treatment option needs to be determined, then the plan should state possible treatment options to investigate. Once the investigation generates sufficient evidence to justify proceeding with one of the options, the plan should be reformulated (to order the chosen procedure and monitor its results). In both of these contexts (diagnostic and therapeutic), knowledge coupling software can help guide the planning process.

Carelessness with this investigative element of initial planning permits the physician to launch into aggressive pursuit of numerous hypotheses without rational priorities or a clear idea of whether the data sought will truly contribute to decision making (as an example, Dr. Groopman describes a surgeon who can't explain what he expects to learn from an arthroscopy except to say, "'I'll figure it out when I get in there'"[192]). This lack of clarity is unacceptable, given the risk, discomfort and expenses often entailed by data collection after the initial database. Patients should demand that the physician distinguish "nice-to-know" from "need-to-know" data. Knowledge coupling software is enormously useful in this regard. After the software harvests the maximum amount of useful information from the initial database and identifies options worth considering, the knowledge coupling output rationally organizes the options identified with the initial data for and against each option, as described in part VI.C.1 above. In the diagnostic context, for example, knowledge coupling output begins with causes for which the prognosis is bad, the course is rapid and effective treatment is known. These diagnostic options should be a higher priority for investigation than self-limiting or untreatable disorders.

---

192 Groopman J. *What Doctors Think*, note 11 above, pp. 162-63.

Use of knowledge coupling software increasingly will make it possible to distinguish between two situations: those where a cluster of simple observations generate sufficient data for decision making vs. those where a costly or invasive procedure is necessary for an informed decision. The latter occurs when such a procedure can be expected to clearly resolve a "need-to-know" issue and alternative approaches would leave uncertainty. Without reliable knowledge coupling to aid in planning, physicians too often confuse these two situations. This confusion is especially dangerous in fee-for-service environments, where providers benefit financially from ordering elaborate and costly procedures. Even where physician reimbursement is structured to avoid direct financial gain, the academic-industrial complex in medicine fosters confusion. A tendency exists to unrealistically attribute diagnostic or therapeutic power to that which is highly technical, expensive, sophisticated or innovative. The most cost-effective tests, procedures, drugs and devices can easily be overlooked for no good reason.

The final element of initial planning is identifying complications to watch for. Careful initial plans should create alertness to early signs of foreseeable complications. For example, patients with infectious mononucleosis can on very rare occasions develop respiratory failure or rupture a spleen. If this possibility is anticipated, then the physician caring for such a patient will pay more attention to the patient's remarks about breathing difficulty, and will check the patient's spleen in follow-up visits. Too often, emergencies occur because no one thought to check for signals given by the patient long before the crisis erupted.

Formulating initial plans represents a crucial opportunity for practitioners to communicate their thought processes to each other and the patient. And making those thought processes clear, structured and explicit is critical to coordination and follow-through. This need—and the failure of current EHRs to satisfy it—were emphasized repeatedly at the Meaningful Use Workgroup hearing discussed above. One witness testified, for example, that in "most EHRs, ... people tend not to document their thought process" because "there's no good place" to do so. These records may be voluminous, "but there isn't the thing that you really care about, which is, this is what I thought. This is what I think it is, and this is what I want to do next. That's evaporated."[193] Failure to communicate thought processes can lead to enormous waste. As another hearing witness testified about referrals to specialists, failure to specify the reason for referral (a commonplace occurrence) means that specialists often "don't have a clue" about what is expected from them. A referral should communicate "one, why is the referral being done. Two, what has been done previously that might be relevant ... so

193 Testimony of Rushika Fernandpulle. See the hearing transcript (note 163 above) at pp. 26-27. See also pp. 16, 18, 23, 36-37, 39, 43, 57, 62, 71, 75 for further discussion of the importance of practitioners' communicating their thought processes.

the specialist doesn't have to say, I give up. Let me just order everything and do everything in the hopes that maybe, you know, one of my darts will hit the dartboard." Enforcing the POMR standard of care would remedy these failings.

Now we turn to the fourth phase of medical action, the crucial stage of follow-up, feedback and corrective action.

4. Progress notes

The uncertainties inherent in complex biologic systems mean that initial plans routinely miss their mark. This reality demands a mechanism for ongoing feedback and adjustment on each plan for each problem. Structured progress notes create the required mechanism.[194]

A core principle of the POMR standard is that all practitioners must conceive and label all progress notes by the problem to which they relate. This principle departs from traditional practice in two ways. First, the scope and structure of traditional physician notes is left to the judgment of physicians. Second, progress notes traditionally are grouped by source, such as a primary care physician, interns, residents, radiologist and pathologist reports, other consulting specialists, nurses, physical therapists, social workers, operative notes and other sources. We consider both of these practices in turn.

First, complex patients typically have multiple problems, some of which are clearly interrelated—for example, a patient with renal failure, congestive heart failure, chronic obstructive lung disease and hypertension. The temptation is to write a single note analyzing these problems together. But the apparent efficiency of doing so is illusory. The parameters required to assess these different problems and the issues they present for analysis are not identical. Without problem-oriented notes, crucial elements are easily overlooked, assessments degenerate to vague generalities like "doing well" or "situation not improving," and needed follow-up is less likely to occur. Moreover, failure to correlate progress notes with specific problems makes it difficult for anyone reviewing the record to understand development of the problem, the significance of data and the purpose of tests and procedures described in the notes.

Second, source-oriented progress notes are not organized by patient needs. Instead, they are organized by institutional needs—the sources of the notes. This practice is completely inconsistent with any concept of "patient-centered" or "consumer-driven" care. To be enforced, that concept must become operational in the structure of a unitary medical record to which all providers contribute. All practitioners must conceive their actions in relation to a specific problem on

---

194 This section draws on *Knowledge Coupling*, note 2 above, pp. 113-40.

the *patient's* problem list, and label their progress notes accordingly. Initial plans are similarly problem-oriented, which facilitates writing notes with the initial plan clearly in mind. In this way, practitioners occupying very different roles find themselves working together on the patient's problems in a unified way over time.

Some readers might object that the problem-oriented structure could hinder consideration of interrelationships among problems. Just the opposite is the case. Simply by examining the complete problem list and the sequential notes on each problem, a practitioner working on any one problem can consider the whole patient and interrelationships among problems in a systematic way. This is far more difficult without a problem-oriented record of care. Just as the unaided mind requires knowledge coupling software to integrate patient data with medical knowledge, so the mind requires the problem-oriented medical record to achieve an integrated view of the patient.[195]

As with initial plans, it is not enough for progress notes to be labeled by the problem to which they relate. Their internal structure should include at least the following elements, based on parameters from the initial plan:

- *"Subjective"* data (the patient's own statements of symptoms and progress)

- *"Objective"* data (lab data and physical findings)

- *Assessment* (e.g., a nurse's judgment of the degree of disability, a physician's judgment of whether his diagnostic hypothesis is supported by current data, an evaluation of a treatment's success)

- *Plan* (modifications in diagnostic or therapeutic action)

Progress notes with these four elements (summarized with the acronym "SOAP") are in common use. The order of these elements is significant. "Subjective" data should come first, "to ensure that the patient's point of view is taken into consideration at the outset—a consideration that is seriously neglected by many physicians."[196]   The labels "subjective" and "objective," however, have been criticized. Their connotations are "ironically at odds with" the original "intent to give both status and priority to the voice of the patient. ... Labeling what patients

---

195 For further discussion of the utility of the POMR, see the articles cited by the Institute of Medicine's *The Computer-Based Patient Record*, note 157 above, and the following: Comments on the POMR. In Driggs MF ed. *Problem-directed and medical information systems.* New York: Inter-Continental Medical Book Corporation, 1974; Bartholomew K, note 64 above, pp. 248-77; Gambert S. "A Problem List for Diagnosis." *Clinical Geriatrics*, 10:10, pp. 15-16 (October 2002); Savage P. "A book that changed my practice," BMJ 2001;322:275 (3 February).

196 Weed, LL., *Medical Records, Medical Education and Patient Care*, note 2 above, p. 50.

say as 'subjective' and what physicians and laboratories find as 'objective' tends to minimize the reality of the patient's world and exaggerate the reality of the physician's."[197] We agree with this criticism, and accordingly would replace "Subjective" and "Objective" with "Symptomatic findings" and "Other findings." Those terms fit the well-established "SOAP" acronym.[198]

Often the above four elements are usefully supplemented with others, such as notes of consulting specialists, or a section on medications. Most important, it is typically necessary to include flowsheets (see below).

The internal structure of progress notes continually reminds practitioners to think systematically about the patient's problems, and it provides evidence of whether they have done so. A complete discussion is beyond the scope of this book. The following points, however, are important to understand.

As noted, progress notes should begin with subjective data because progress should be assessed from the patient's point of view. Practitioners should be alert to discrepancies between subjective and objective data (for example, where the patient does not feel better when lab results show improvement). These discrepancies may signal an error in data or misstatement of the patient's problem.

In the objective data section, physicians tend to omit physical findings and emphasize laboratory data. For example, it is not unusual to find detailed discussion of an X-ray and no mention of how the patient coughs or the quantity and character of the sputum. This kind of omission should be noticed and remedied.

In complex cases, objective data typically need to be organized into flowsheets. Flowsheets reveal patterns and interrelationships over time with multiple variables involving physical findings, vital signs, laboratory values, medications and other intakes and outputs. Electronic medical records greatly facilitate creation of flowsheets. Their utility is determined by the choice of variables to include, the choice of time intervals for measurement, and the care with which the data are recorded, monitored and acted upon. Each value entered in a flowsheet should

---

197 Donnelly W, Brauner J. Why SOAP is Bad for the Medical Record, *Arch Intern Med* 152:481-484 (March 1992), pp. 481, 483, available at http://archinte.ama-assn.org/cgi/reprint/152/3/481?ijkey=edec87ce438a54a0449cc46b91a129a13104c06b.

198 Drs. Donnelly and Brauner recommend the terms "History" and "Observations" (p. 483). (See also their discussion of the historical usage of the terms "symptoms" and "signs" in relation to the distinction between information and inference.) We do not think the term "History" works well in progress notes, because it suggests "History of Present Illness" or perhaps "Family History" (other possible terms are "Narrative" or "Story"). As an alternative to "Objective," the term "Observations" suggests personal observations as distinguished from test results and other findings. Accordingly, we prefer the terms "Symptomatic findings" and "Other findings." This is an issue to be resolved by an appropriate standards setting organization.

be compared with preceding values, to observe the rate of change. The greater the rate of change, the more frequently the value should be checked, and the sooner the responsible provider should be notified.

This basic principle about monitoring the rate of change applies not just to flowsheet data but to any objective and subjective data collected over time. Recall our earlier discussions about setting parameters and watching for complications. Patients and their families should be educated about the significance of the data collected, the potential for error in provider judgments and the need to monitor the data as feedback on those judgments. Patients and their families are often well positioned to judge the rate of change in parameters and alert providers. In this regard, patients should think of themselves as the most important provider of their own care. In one case, for example, a patient with a sore throat, fever and malaise noted that what seemed like a small, harmless rash suddenly started to spread—a parameter undergoing a rapid rate of change. She notified no one because a physician had told her she was doing fine and he would see her the next day. The next day never came for her, and a meningococcemia the physician did not foresee took over. It could have been treated earlier and probably successfully if she had been taught to understand the significance of rapidly changing parameters, no matter what they are.

Along with problem lists, the most widely used component of the POMR is progress notes in the "SOAP" format. But the SOAP format for progress notes is usually followed more as a convenience than as a standard or discipline. In contrast, when SOAP notes are titled by the problem to which they relate on a complete list of well-defined patient problems, the notes then become part of a disciplined process of feedback and corrective action. But this rarely occurs. The reality is that POMR standards have been honored as much in the breach as the observance. Physicians use components of the POMR selectively, at their convenience, and without the rigor that patients need.

D. Further perspectives on the POMR

1. Criticisms of the POMR

First developed in the late 1950s, the POMR (or some elements) experienced widespread acceptance once it become prominent in the late 1960's and early 1970's. It also encountered some objections, and variations on the POMR have been suggested. A complete discussion is beyond the scope of this book, but we can address several points here.

One objection was that the problem list, by dividing up the patient's medical situation into separate problems, leads to fragmented care. The most extreme statement of this view was that the POMR permits each specialist to consider only the problem pertaining to his specialty and then "depart—without having to be exposed to or become aware of any problems beyond the boundaries of that specialty."[199] Precisely the opposite is the case. The POMR standard demands that planning for each problem take into account the patient's other problems and life situation. See parts VI.C.1 and 3. This standard of care is unattainable without the discipline of maintaining a complete problem list and together with a patient profile. Stated differently, that discipline creates a basis for holding accountable practitioners who fail to take into account the patient's total needs. The same article implicitly recognized this accountability, referring to the patient profile as one of the "major virtues" of the POMR: "By demanding a description of the patient's life style in conjunction with the patient's medical data, the new 'Patient Profile' is an important mechanism for calling attention to the total situation about which a good physician should be informed"—and for calling attention to a practitioner who ignores the total situation.[200]

A related objection is that labeling all plans and progress notes by the problem to which each relates causes difficulties when problems are interrelated and the practitioner wishes to view all the related data together, organized chronologically. There are several responses to this concern. First, plans and progress notes for one problem can cross-reference another problem, based on specific interrelationships of concern. Second, the same data item can be entered under more than one problem (each entry should include a problem-specific assessment of the data item for *that* problem). Third, electronic records can be designed to permit chronological views of data from two or more problems. Indeed, the problem-oriented structure maximizes flexibility in this regard, because the user can select the problems for which data would be combined and displayed chronologically.[201]

Knowledge coupling software directly addresses another criticism of the POMR: that "there are no guidelines" for determining what data points are sufficient to confirm a hypothesis.[202] This criticism was an overstatement at the time, for in many cases a hypothesis can be confirmed based on available data in light of commonly known and accepted guidance from the medical literature

199 Feinstein A., The Problems of the Problem_Oriented Medical Record. *Annals Int. Med.*,78-751-762 (May 1973), pp. 756-57.

200 *Ibid.*, p. 754.

201 See Bainbridge M., et al. The Problem-Oriented Medical Record – just a little more structure to help the world go round?, Clinical Computing Special Interest Group of the PHCSG, available at www.phcsg.org/main/pastconf/camb96/mikey.htm.

202 Goldfinger, S. The Problem-Oriented Record: A Critique from a Believer. *New Eng. J. Med.*, 288(12):606-608 (March 22, 1973).

(the Addison's disease case in part II.A is an example). In any event, this difficulty greatly diminishes with the use of knowledge coupling software. The user employs the software to locate the most relevant available guidelines from the literature. No longer must clinicians and their patients settle for limited personal knowledge of that literature. The literature may or may not clarify what data points are sufficient to confirm a hypothesis, depending on whether or not a medical consensus exists on the specific point in question. Regardless, the knowledge coupling software exposes the existence or lack of consensus and its basis. That medical knowledge is then continuously tested against reality by patients, practitioners and researchers who examine the software's output.

A more recent observer has argued that the computerized POMR needs "an automated method for organizing patient data around medical problems identified from clinical documents" and that this should be accomplished by "natural language processing (NLP) to automatically identify and extract clinical problems, their associated findings, and attributes that are classifiable along four dimensions (axes): time, space, existence, and causality."[203] Knowledge coupling software accomplishes the goal of "organizing patient data around medical problems identified from clinical documents," and it does so without the pitfalls of natural language processing (which permits undefined, uncontrolled inputs —natural language—from the physician's unaided mind).

2. *The POMR and its integration with knowledge coupling from an IT perspective*

Dr. Ken Bartholomew has provided an operational description of the PKC POMR system as he used it in conjunction with knowledge coupling software. Using actual patient encounters as examples, he describes improvements and efficiencies he experienced, both clinically and administratively. One patient he describes, for example, had 21 problems on her problem list, with complete information on each problem arranged in outline form under predefined headings, available by clicking on the problem number/title. The course of each of these problems could be "followed almost at a glance instead of having to page through all of this patient's laboratory and progress note data." One problem, for example, atrial fibrillation, had 34 entries, seven levels deep, including lab tests of multiple types, all readily viewable in different contexts. Any lab test can be retrieved in seconds, with the results displayed chronologically in flowsheet format, regardless of the problem for which the test was ordered. This display of the results further enables the user to go back into the chart at the point where

---

203 Bashyam V. et al, Problem-Centric Organization and Visualization of Patient Imaging and Clinical Data," *RadioGraphics* 2009; 29:331–343.

the test was entered, permitting review of not only the lab value or result but also the time it was performed, the problem for which it was ordered and the reason for the order. Similarly, the chronology and basis of problem definition and redefinition over time are clear. The record format is flexible in both data entry and display, so that specific levels and headings can be bypassed if not relevant. The record system's design was simple and intuitive, enabling its implementation without any computer-literate staff.[204]

These capabilities are partially inherent in the POMR standard, partially the result of the software's speed and ease of use, and partially the result of how medical knowledge was represented in the system. The last factor is what we briefly discuss here, in extremely simplified form.

Medical knowledge can be conceptualized as a set of entities and properties of those entities. Entities include such items as diagnoses, lab tests, medications, and clinical imaging. Entities are stored in a separate file, the medical entity list. Each entity has a property list. Properties are important information about an entity. A medication entity, for example, has properties such as the generic name, synonyms, drug class, actions, warnings, contraindications, dosage, and much other information.

The entity and property lists enable great flexibility and efficiency in data retrievals, both within and across individual patient records, as Dr. Bartholomew describes in some detail. But much more resides in the underlying knowledge net from which entity and property lists can be derived. Specifically, the knowledge net associates each relationship between a pair of entities with two types of classifying and conditioning information: (1) the relation type or class, and (2) textual commentary explaining the entity relationship. The knowledge net holding this information is used to build Couplers, as we further discuss at the end of Part VII.B.2.

The flexibility of the knowledge net enables medical knowledge to be organized, searched and retrieved in a problem-oriented manner. This is not possible with the medical literature. The knowledge net was built by exploring the medical literature with reference to specific problems not as ultimately analyzed by physicians but as initially presented by patients (e.g. unexplained symptoms for diagnosis, complex conditions for management). In this way,

---

204 See pages 248-77 of Dr. Bartholomew's chapter in *Knowledge Coupling*, note 2 above (see 251-54 for the particular patient discussed above). The programming to create both the POMR and knowledge coupling tools was done by Richard Hertzberg, whose work brought to life many of the concepts discussed in this book.

precisely relevant information is extracted from the medical literature, distilled, and presented to users in maximally usable form.[205]

3. Resistance to the POMR

The real question to be raised about the POMR does not involve specific criticisms like those discussed in part VI.D.1. The real question is why the POMR was never fully embraced as a standard of care for medical practice, indeed, why its usage has declined since it first became widespread. The central reason, we believe, is that the disciplines the POMR imposes are alien to the culture of medicine. Notwithstanding the increasing use of EHRs, the culture of medicine is still rooted in World 2 (see the text at notes 108-109 above), where provider judgments reign, where the unaided mind determines the content of EHRs, where unexamined habits determine the organization of EHRs, where a transparent, external infrastructure essential for accountability and patient autonomy is lacking.

Changing the culture of medicine depends on the POMR. Its common-sense, intuitive structure is one that everyone can readily understand and use. At the same time, it is scientifically rigorous and clinically effective. Together with knowledge coupling standards and tools, EHRs adhering to the POMR standard establish an essential architecture for a system in which consumers and expert practitioners can jointly play their respective roles, subject to feedback and continuous improvement.[206]

---

205 For further discussion, see Knowledge Coupling, note 2 above, pp. 149-53, 250-58; and PKC Corporation, and "A Problem-Oriented Approach to the Computerized Patient Record (1998), at http://www.pkc.com/papers/pomr.pdf.

206 Dr. Ken Bartholomew has described how the simplicity of the DOS-based PKC electronic POMR enabled him to adopt it in his office in the late 1980s without any computer literate staff. *Knowledge Coupling*, note 2 above, p. 254. For a careful discussion of how the POMR fosters quality improvement, see Graves S. Better Records: First Step to Better Quality. *Modern Hospital*, 116:105-108 (1971), reprinted in *Applying the Problem-Oriented System*, note 174 above, pp. 266-71. By comparison, current discussions of health policy in general and health IT in particular largely overlook or even reject the need for basic standards of data organization in medical records. See for example Report of the President's Council of Advisors on Science and Technology (PCAST), *Realizing the Full Potential of Health Information Technology: The Path Forward* (December 2010), http://www.whitehouse.gov/sites/default/files/microsites/ostp/pcast-health-it-report.pdf. The PCAST report states, "any attempt to create a national health IT ecosystem based on standardized record formats is doomed to failure" (p. 39). The PCAST report does not consider the possibility that standardized record formats could be a part of the "simple rules" essential to creating a complex adaptive system for health care (see part above). For comments (including the authors') on the PCAST report submitted to the Office of the National Coordinator for Health IT, see www.regulations.gov/#!docketDetail;dct=FR+PR+N+O+SR;rpp=10;so=DESC;sb=postedDate;po=0;D=HHS-OS-2010-0030

Building the infrastructure and changing the culture of medicine cannot be left to the medical profession alone. Leaders outside the profession, and especially the general public, need to understand the transformation that is possible. But writings like this book will not make that happen. A recurring pattern in the history of medicine is the persistence of ineffective or harmful practices, and resistance to needed innovations. What is needed to change that pattern is public understanding of why the status quo is bankrupt, a shared vision of an alternative, and an external compulsion to change. What is needed is something like what happened to the American auto industry in the 1980s and 1990s. There, Edwards Deming (exiled to Japan) developed an alternative to the status quo, Japanese manufacturers created a working model of what could be achieved and exported that model to the U.S., the public used its buying power, and the industry was forced to change under threat of bankruptcy.

This kind of market competition cannot yet happen to the same extent in medicine, because it is blocked by the medical profession's monopoly (see part VIII.B below). But even within that current legal framework, the opportunity exists for communities to create large-scale working models of much of the transformation that is needed. If that happens, then the culture of medicine can evolve in that direction, and the new infrastructure of tools can be built. But that will not be enough.

Leaders must begin to conceive institutional arrangements for developing and enforcing standards of care for managing clinical information, just as the domain of commerce has institutional arrangements (e.g., the Financial Accounting Standards Board, the auditing profession) to develop and enforce standards of care for managing financial information. It does little good to subsidize the purchase of EHRs if their inputs are not guided and defined by knowledge coupling software compatible with the EHR design. It does little good to equip practitioners with knowledge coupling software if they are left free to exercise judgment on when to use the software or what data to collect. It does little good to design interoperable EHRs for exchanging patient data if the design does not also organize the data for coordinated care of multiple problems by multiple practitioners over time. It does little good for multiple EHR vendors to separately design such EHRs if variations reduce interoperability and ready comprehension by all.

Finally, legal reforms and institutional arrangements are needed for training and credentialing individual providers and accrediting institutional providers. As we shall see in part VIII, it does little good to rebuild the intellectual infrastructure and standards of practice for health care, if educational and credentialing institutions are constantly feeding the system with autonomous physician experts whose credentials block competition by others better prepared to function within a disciplined system of care.

Before we examine training and credentialing, we need to further discuss the nature of the medical knowledge that practitioners are expected to apply.

VII.
The Gap Between Medical Knowledge and Individual Patients

She could not eat or sleep, grew visibly thinner, coughed, and, as the doctors made them feel, was in danger. They could not think of anything but how to help her. Doctors came to see her singly and in consultation, talked much in French, German and Latin, blamed one another, and prescribed a great variety of medicines for all the diseases known to them, but the simple idea never occurred to any of them that they could not know the disease Natásha was suffering from, as no disease suffered by a live man can be known, for every living person has his own peculiarities and always has his own peculiar, personal, novel, complicated disease, unknown to medicine—not a disease of the lungs, liver, skin, heart, nerves and so on mentioned in the medical books, but a disease consisting of one of the innumerable combinations of the maladies of those organs.

— *Leo Tolstoy*[207]

And generally, let this be a rule, that all partitions of knowledge be accepted rather for lines and veins than for sections and separations; and that the continuance and entireness of knowledge be preserved. For the contrary hereof hath made particular sciences to become barren, shallow, and erroneous, while they have not been maintained from the common fountain.

— *Francis Bacon*[208]

---

207 Tolstoy L. *War and Peace* (1869), Book Nine, Chapter 16 (Maude trans.). Tolstoy's passage goes on to describe why physicians have difficulty perceiving disease as "one of the innumerable combinations" of the maladies of multiple organs: "This simple thought could not occur to the doctors because, … above all, … they saw that they were really useful … They satisfied that eternal human need for hope of relief, for sympathy, and that something should be done, which is felt by those who are suffering." This is one reason why the relationship between practitioner and patient may itself be therapeutic, as we have discussed (part IV.G.4) but may also limit perception. The eternal human need for hope of relief reinforces the human mind's eternal need to simplify complex realities.

208 Bacon F. *The Advancement of Learning*, IX(1), at http://www.fullbooks.com/The-Advancement-of-Learning2.html

Medical knowledge is itself an element of the health care system. Like other elements, medical knowledge is distorted by failure to migrate from the realm of subjective, personal knowledge to the realm of objective knowledge, from knowledge as it exists in the mind to its independent existence in external information tools.[209] The distortion occurs in the *content* of medical knowledge, in its *organization*, and in its *capacity for growth.*

First, the content of medical knowledge is oriented towards resemblances, not differences, among individuals. Yet, the differences must be taken into account for sound decision making, especially with chronic disease. Thus, individual heterogeneity and uniqueness, no less than patterns of resemblance across populations, must become the subject matter of medical knowledge.

Second, the health care system fails to organize medical knowledge for solving the problems of unique patients, just as the system fails to organize health care providers for delivering patient-centered care. Care is thus fragmented intellectually as well as institutionally. Rather than being oriented towards patient needs, knowledge is organized for comprehension by the unaided minds of physicians. Medical specialties, for example, are defined by body system. That narrow focus reduces the burden of comprehension, but it fails to cope with the reality that patient problems normally implicate multiple body systems. Similarly, the population-based content of medical knowledge is easier for the mind to comprehend than detailed data about individual variation.

Third, the health care system fails to enforce the scientific standards and tools essential to the growth of reliable medical knowledge. Existing "knowledge" is not just incomplete but in part is simply wrong. As with other areas of science, medical knowledge is only a provisional approximation of reality. Practitioners, patients and researchers must constantly test medical knowledge against reality. In caregiving, that testing process demands taking into account all potentially relevant knowledge and patient-specific data at the outset of care, and then carefully monitoring and adjusting whatever course of action is chosen. In clinical research, that testing process demands continuously harvesting feedback on knowledge by examining meticulous records of what happens when knowledge is applied.

From this point of view, the following considers different forms of medical knowledge, their relation to patient-specific data and how these issues relate to evidence-based medicine, medical practice, and research.

---

209 Recall Popper's distinction between World 2 and World 3 (see note 108), discussed in part V.A.1.

A. General knowledge and the individual patient

1. *Two forms of medical knowledge*

Conceiving medical knowledge as generalizations about populations of individuals is not complete. Medical decision making routinely demands taking into account individual variations from what population-based knowledge leads us to expect.

a. *Population-based knowledge*

Consider first what is meant by the population-based concept of medical knowledge. Some of the great advances in medical science are applicable to large populations without regard to variations among individuals. Salk's development of a polio vaccine, for example, involved a single therapeutic agent that prevents polio in virtually everyone. In that context, differences among individuals have no significance except in the very few cases where the vaccine may not be safe or effective. Similarly, even in contexts where individual variations have critical and pervasive significance, individual needs cannot be addressed without applying general principles of pathophysiology applicable to large populations. All diabetics, for example, despite their enormous variability, have in common some dysfunction in hormonal regulation of blood glucose levels. Indeed, diabetes is *defined* in those terms. Medical knowledge is thus naturally conceived as applicable to large populations.

This population-based concept of medical knowledge also applies to variations within a large population when multiple individuals with a particular variation or set of variations in common are grouped into a definable subpopulation. For example, the population of diabetics can be grouped into myriad subpopulations, ranging from extremely broad groupings (Type I or Type II diabetics) to narrower ones (Type I diabetics with chronic renal insufficiency and cardiovascular disease).

Population-based knowledge may be either explanatory (principles of pathophysiology) or descriptive (statistical information without an explanation for what is described). In either case, population-based knowledge is fallible. Consider, for example, clinical trial results showing statistically significant favorable outcomes for a drug in a randomized population of individuals with a given disease and without co-morbidities. The outcome data are descriptive; they do not explain why the drug is successful for some individuals and not others in the clinical trial population. Nor do outcome data explain when the drug is appropriate for individuals with co-morbidities or other differences from the clinical trial population. Nor do outcome data explain when off-label use of the drug is appropriate. Pathophysiologic explanations to answer these questions may be offered. But the answers must be tested against the results of actual use with patients. And those results will not yield trustworthy feedback without meticulous medical records providing detailed data about the patients receiving the drug.

b. *Knowledge about individual variation*

Population-based knowledge as just described has become extraordinarily voluminous and complex. But a further category of medical knowledge exists— medical knowledge about variations at the individual level. This occurs with individuals who seem anomalous in some way, that is, whose characteristics depart unexpectedly from some relevant subpopulation. Such knowledge often takes the form of case reports such as the *New England Journal* article we discussed in part II.A, where the patient's presentation of Addison's disease was described as atypical. In addition to such reports, medical knowledge of variations at the individual level could, in principle, take the form of patient data in medical records. But those data are not accessible for research purposes in the way that published case reports are accessible, and therefore cannot be considered part of the body of medical knowledge (although that could change, as discussed below). By comparison, genomic and proteomic information about individuals may become accessible for research purposes and therefore become part of the body of medical knowledge.

Variations at the individual level are usually viewed as exceptions from the norm. The norm, we are taught, is "the textbook case," the model that other cases are expected to resemble. Yet, "the textbook case is so rare that everyone runs to look at it in the medical center when it is found," as Dr. Ken Bartholomew has observed. In reality, the textbook case is the exception, and variations from it are the norm. "Patient presentations are not one textbook scenario but thousands of similar, yet unique, combinations of presentations that our experience enables us to categorize." The dilemma is that *personal* experience is limited, and the mind categorizes even that limited experience simplistically. The textbook case thus becomes "a self-fulfilling prophecy"; unexpected variations from it are not searched for or recognized.[210] The Addison's disease case study discussed above illustrates this phenomenon.

Individual case reports are important to the progress of medical science. Reports of variations from known patterns can lead to uncovering new diseases, rare manifestations of known diseases, drug side effects, and new understanding

210 Bartholomew K. "The Perspective of a Practitioner," in Knowledge Coupling, note 2 above, p. 240.

of disease mechanisms.[211] But poor feedback mechanisms block this progress at multiple levels. The unaided mind, following textbook knowledge, may not even recognize variations; or variations may be misclassified; or medical records may be too incomplete and unstructured to generate adequate case reports; or published case reports may be overlooked by practitioners or patients when those reports are directly relevant.

To reiterate, no practitioner can be aware of all the known patterns to consider, much less variations from those patterns. Pattern recognition in the face of such complexity requires tools external to the mind. Once those tools are employed, the mind develops new perceptions of both the patterns and the individuals with whom the patterns are compared. The next section describes those new perceptions.

2. The concept of individual uniqueness

The dilemma faced by practitioners and researchers is that known patterns are rough generalizations about large populations, and as such are usually an imperfect fit with unique individuals. Every individual is a unique combination of myriad similarities to and differences from other individuals. What constitutes a similarity or difference depends on the particular diagnostic or therapeutic context. The similarities mean that different individuals can be medically classified together in the same category— a trait or set of traits in common with other individuals. The differences mean that various individuals classified in the same category are nevertheless different from each other in various respects that may provide different keys to solving the medical problem they seem to have in common.[212]

The similarities and differences arise initially from each individual's unique genetic heritage and unique developmental history. Each individual is a recombination of pre-existing biological elements, which are built into an enormously complex set of interconnected structures and interacting processes. The recombination of elements is not static but continuously evolving, subject to both internal and external forces. An important internal force is the human body's extraordinary capacity for self-regulation (known as homeostasis) and self-repair. As a result, the normal physiology of healthy persons become increasingly differentiated over time.

---

211 Vandenbroucke J. In Defense of Case Reports and Case Series. 2001. *Annals of Internal Medicine*. 134:330-334 (Feb. 20, 2001).

212 The following discussion draws heavily on Weed, CC. *The Philosophy, Use and Interpretation of Knowledge Couplers*, note 2 above.

This complexity increases by orders of magnitude when normal physiology is disrupted by pathophysiologic processes, psychological processes, the physical environment, the social environment and medical interventions. Some aspects, such as newly evolved pathogens or unidentified disease processes, may be unknown to medical science. Thus a person's total medical condition can be regarded as a single, aggregate, new disease entity, described by Tolstoy as that person's "own peculiar, personal, novel, complicated disease, unknown to medicine."

The interacting elements introduce multiple layers of complexity and disruption. As stated by Dickinson Richards, in words that apply both to human physiology and its external environment:

> Man's power became ever greater, but this curiously made matters worse not better, because his power became too great for his understanding, and moved even further beyond his awareness of consequences. ... Man's unbridled use of his technological armament throws whole segments of the natural order out of balance, with the full meaning of this obscure, the outcome unknown. [213]

In short, each person's illness will be a unique course of events, never precisely reproduced in any other person. Chronic illness in particular becomes highly personalized in this way. Consequently, when different individuals are labeled with the same illness, their medical condition and therapeutic needs may in fact differ radically. Diagnosis and treatment of each person's illness must take into account the myriad resemblances to and differences from many other persons' experiences of the "same" illness. Doing so far exceeds the capacity of the human mind.

None of these points are surprising. Indeed, they are consistent with intuition, common experience and basic scientific knowledge. But without the tools needed to act on these points, their implications elude us.

B. Some implications

1. The gap between evidence-based medicine and individual patient needs

... we must bring men to particulars, and their regular series and order, and they must for a while renounce their notions and begin to form an acquaintance with things.

— Francis Bacon[214]

---

213 Richards D. "Hippocrates and History: The Arrogance of Humanism," *Hippocrates Revisited*, note 54 above, pp. 25, 26.

214 Bacon F. *Novum Organon* (1620), Aphorism No. 36. See note 1 above. The qualification "for a while" shows the sophistication of Bacon's thought. He recognized that we cannot form

For centuries an unresolved debate has been carried on in medicine about the meaning of an individual patient's risk[215] and the concepts of induction and probability as applied in patient care.[216] During the past two decades the debate has provided the framework for critiques of managed care (in the U.S.) and evidence-based medicine (EBM).

"EBM and managed care share a common ethical and epistemologic focus on outcomes measured across populations."[217] Both epistemologically and ethically, this focus is misplaced in the context of patient care. As Chris Weed has observed, statistical information about population outcomes answers questions that patients and their practitioners do not ask:

> Statistical answers are rationally useful only when one is interested not in individual cases but in regularities occurring in large numbers of cases. In other words, the patient is not in the position of a gambling casino. He or she is not in a position to say that if money is lost to the customers one day (the patient's illness is misdiagnosed or mismanaged), the odds are that it will be recovered several times over within a week. The patient may in a very real sense be "open for business" only for that day.[218]

Epistemologically, outcomes measured across populations do not permit us to know the expected outcome for an individual who differs in relevant respects from the measured population—and relevant differences are the norm, not the exception. Ethically, population-based decision making rests on an "assumption that outcomes faced by individual persons can offset each other," as Asch and Hershey observe. That assumption "effaces the moral distinction between those persons." Outcomes among population members can be permitted to offset each

---

a wholly objective "acquaintance with things," because inevitably we have some preconceived "notions" that shape and select what we observe. Nevertheless, we must "begin" to form an independent acquaintance of things, initially attempting to renounce our notions so that after a while we may redefine and test them. See also Zagorin P. Francis Bacon's concept of objectivity and the idols of the mind, *BJHS*, 2001, 34, 379-393 (criticizing "the mistaken image we still have of Bacon as a pure empiricist who wished to divorce science from theories, hypotheses and interpretations," p. 391).

215 Goodman S. Probability at the bedside: the knowing of chances or the chances of knowing? *Ann Intern Med* 1999;130:604-606.

216 Hanckel F. The problem of induction in clinical decision making. *Medical Decision Making.* 1984;4:59-68.

217 Tonelli M. The Philosophical Limits of Evidence-Based Medicine. *Academic Medicine,* 1998; 73: 1234-1240 (p. 1238).

218 Weed CC. *The Philosophy, Use and Interpretation of Knowledge Couplers,* note 2 above, p. 4. The quoted statement, written in 1982, predated the rise of managed care and evidence-based medicine, but it articulated the reason why physicians and patients distrusted those developments.

other in veterinary care for livestock herds, but not in health care for human beings.[219]

A central reason for the population perspective is that so much of medical care is paid for by third parties. A third party payer views cost-effectiveness in relation to the entire covered population. But individuals within that population view cost-effectiveness in relation to their individual needs, and they purchase health coverage (both group and individual) on that basis. The benefit of that bargain is denied to its intended beneficiaries when their individual needs are not served.

Therefore, in optimizing decisions for individuals, the uniqueness of each individual must be rigorously taken into account. This reality is now invariably acknowledged by evidence-based medicine proponents. But they underestimate the extent of individual uniqueness within populations, and fail to define a rigorous, systematic approach for taking that uniqueness into account. For example, one authoritative statement of EBM principles explains: "we must remember that recommendations can be made only for average patients, and the circumstances and values of the patient before us differ."[220] This seems to imply that average patients are medically similar, differing only in non-medical circumstances and values, and therefore that medical recommendations can apply across a population, subject only to individual adjustments for non-medical differences. The reality, however, is that virtually all individuals differ *medically* from the average. That is, they differ not just in their circumstances and values but in their medical characteristics bearing on the problem presented. The details of those differences, not population averages, must be the start and end points of individual decision making. Averages are useful, if at all, only for clues about which details are the highest priority for analysis.

Misconceiving individual variations as exceptions to population-based rules perverts the core element of evidence-based medicine, its "hierarchy of evidence." At the top of this hierarchy are randomized clinical trials (RCTs). Randomization deliberately excludes most individual variations, even those (such as co-morbidities) manifestly relevant to individual decision making. Other forms of population-based evidence, such as large observational studies and systematic reviews, similarly exclude or overlook potentially relevant data about individual variation. Evidence-based medicine thus directs clinicians to

---

219 Asch D, Hershey J. Why some health policies don't make sense at the bedside. *Ann Intern Med* 1995; 222:846-850 (p. 848).

220 Guyon G. et al. (for the Evidence-Based Medicine Working Group). "Users' Guides to the Medical Literature. XXV. Evidence-Based Medicine: Principles for Applying the Users' Guides to Patient Care. " *JAMA* 284:10; 1290-1296 (Sep. 13, 2000, p. 1294)

look first to population-based general rules and then to consider individual variations merely as exceptions to those rules.

This hierarchy is upside down. Knowledge about large populations is useless, indeed misleading, until other, more individually applicable knowledge is first taken into account. Thus the *sequence* in which evidence is considered is crucial. Recall from the Addison's disease case study in Part II.A how the physicians first looked for diagnoses thought to be common in the population of people suffering from severe fatigue, despite details about their patient revealing her to be quite unlike that large population and very much like the small subpopulation of people with Addison's disease. Recall further how the article characterized the patient's presentation of the disease as atypical, when in reality her presentation should have been seen as one of many possible expected variations within recognizable patterns of the disease. This example illustrates how the population-based perspective suppresses awareness of individual variation, and inhibits clinicians from taking into account patient-specific details.

More complete than this population-based perspective is a perspective that begins and ends with awareness of each patient's uniqueness. Continuing with the Addison's disease example, that disease can be defined in terms of a single abnormality—deficiency in adrenal-cortical hormones. Yet that one element can interact with unique individual physiologies in enormously variable ways. We thus can conceive Addison's disease in either population-based or individualized terms, that is, either (1) the basic element common to the entire population with the disease (the hormone deficiency), or (2) the variable ways in which unique individuals respond to the hormone deficiency and manifest the disease. The second, individualized conception is too detailed to be captured in textbook terms or comprehended by the unaided mind.

These principles apply in the therapeutic as well as diagnostic context.[221] Consider clinical trial results for drug therapy. Such results are typically expressed as "average treatment effects" in the trial population relative to a placebo or alternative therapies. Yet, the average obscures heterogeneous treatment effects within the trial population, not to mention differences between that population

---

221 The utility of these principles varies with the context. For example, in the therapeutic context, the population-based concept of Addison's disease is useful, because most patients with the disease can be successfully treated with simple hormone replacement therapy. In the diagnostic context, the individualized perspective becomes somewhat more important, because Addison's disease manifests itself in variable ways. Yet, Addison's disease should be relatively simple to diagnose, because recognizable patterns of the disease can be ascertained from organized data collection and analysis. Many conditions are much more complex to diagnose or treat, and even simple conditions can become difficult in patients who have co-morbid conditions or other complicating factors.

and the populations that may later use a drug therapy.[222] Thus, for an individual patient considering use of the drug, the population average is much less relevant than a detailed comparison of the patient's medical characteristics with those of two subpopulations: individuals who experienced a favorable outcome and those who experienced an unfavorable outcome. Suppose detailed comparison of careful medical records on the patient and careful records on the clinical trial population reveals that the patient closely resembles the subpopulation with a favorable outcome. In that case, the population average is essentially irrelevant to that patient. Decision making based on large population studies is becoming increasingly pointless now that we can analyze individual variation and small subpopulations at the level of genes and protein molecules.

The primacy of patient-specific evidence does not mean that population-based evidence is useless. On the contrary, once detailed initial data are taken into account, population-based evidence can then provide useful guidance to prioritize investigation. In the diagnostic context, where detailed patient data initially suggest several plausible diagnoses, it is then useful to know which of those possibilities are most common. Other things being equal, a common condition should be a higher priority for investigation than a rare condition. But using population-based knowledge of prevalence to select the highest priority diagnostic possibility is only an intermediate step. The next step is collecting new patient-specific data to confirm or rule out that possibility. Once collected, the new data supersede population-based evidence as a basis for decision.

Similarly, in the treatment context, patient-specific data bearing on suitability of a treatment for an individual patient should normally supersede population-based guidelines about aggregate therapeutic efficacy. Efficacy often varies substantially among individuals within a population, including a randomized population in a clinical trial. That heterogeneity is obscured when population-based therapeutic outcomes are expressed as population averages. Individualized decision making requires taking into account patient-specific information bearing on four dimensions of individual variability:

---

222 See McMurray J, O'Meara E. Treatment of Heart Failure with Spironolactone — Trial and Tribulations, 2004. *New Eng J Med* 351:6; 526-529; Juurlink D et al., Rates of Hyperkalemia After Publication of the Randomized Aldactone Evaluation Study. 2004. *New Eng J Med* 351:6; 543-551. These articles describe a large discrepancy between a favorable clinical trial of a drug for advanced congestive heart failure and unfavorable outcomes associated with increased use of the drug after the trial results were published and disseminated in practice guidelines. The articles analyze a number of foreseeable explanations for this discrepancy, including clear differences between the real-world population receiving the drug and the randomized trial population.

the patient's (1) baseline probability of incurring a disease-related adverse event ("risk without treatment" or "susceptibility/ prognosis"), (2) responsiveness to the treatment, (3) vulnerability to the adverse effects of the treatment, and (4) utilities [personal values and preferences] for different outcomes.[223]

The above discussion suggests that randomized clinical trials in their present form are a poor substitute for rigorous medical practice as a source of evidence to inform decision making. In particular, analysis of drug safety and efficacy could become more accurate, timely, and affordable, if rigor was brought to medical record keeping and coupling of medical knowledge with patient data. In contrast, as Dr. Scott Gottlieb has observed, current regulatory approaches are futile:

> The fundamental problem inside the FDA is … the quality of information on which the FDA can base its evaluations. Today, the data that medical reviewers receive in conjunction with the process for approving new products are from highly structured clinical trials, carried out on homogenous populations of patients that are carefully screened and preselected and then given new drugs under special protocols. There is little chance that such trials will ever provide a complete review of how a new treatment will perform when it is used in much broader populations of patients in real-world clinical settings, where patients do not always take their medicines on time or at all; where patients might have other medical problems or be of advanced age or in frail health; and where they have comorbidities or unusual diets, or they fill prescriptions for medications or dietary supplements that interact with one another, subtly or otherwise. [224]

Dr. Gottlieb goes on to point out that clinical trials large enough for validity are extraordinarily time-consuming and costly, and it is sometimes impossible to recruit patients with the desired characteristics for such trials.

Moreover, as few as one percent of all adverse drug events are estimated to be reported by physicians under the current passive reporting systems.[225] Being dependent on physician initiative and not integrated with medical practice, these

---

223 Kravitz R, Duan N, Braslow J. Evidence-Based Medicine, Heterogeneity of Treatment Effects and the Trouble with Averages. *The Milbank Quarterly*, 2004, 82:4; 661-687 (p. 662); Erratum at http://www.milbank.org/erratum4-4.pdf.

224 Gottlieb S., Opening Pandora's Pillbox: Using Modern Information Tools To Improve Drug Safety. note 142 above, p. 939.

225 *Ibid.*, pp. 939-41.

systems are insufficient for harvesting reliable data about adverse drug events. Instead, that data should be available as a byproduct of the information tools that practitioners and patients use for their own functioning. Regulators and researchers could continuously harvest that data and rapidly identify patterns of adverse drug events.

The population-based perspective distorts not only clinical decision making and quality reporting/research but also concepts of quality control. Consider, for example, the numerous studies documenting large geographic variation in utilization rates of health care services without any corresponding variations in medical needs in the respective geographic areas.[226] These studies raise two basic questions: (1) what utilization rate of the services in question is appropriate, and (2) how can appropriate usage be enforced uniformly? At first glance, these questions may seem readily answerable by population-based analysis. For example, in some cases the answer to the first question is that variations may seem clearly attributable to provider-induced demand (because of correlation between utilization rates and the supply of providers). The answer to the second question might be to counteract provider-induced demand by using evidence-based practice guidelines to restrict provider discretion.

But such conclusions beg the most important question—how do we improve the basis for decision making, so that patient care decisions will be optimal for each patient, regardless of geographic area? Evidence-based practice guidelines derived from large population studies are no answer to this question because they do not take into account relevant, patient-specific details. The only way to take those details into account is to employ external tools designed for selection and analysis of detailed data in light of medical knowledge. If individual decisions are optimized in that manner, and if the personnel, procedures, drugs, devices and facilities used to execute those decisions are reliable, then whatever level of aggregate usage results from those decisions is appropriate, regardless of whether or how usage varies geographically. Consider again the transportation system analogy discussed in part I. If roads and traffic systems are carefully monitored and-maintained in good working order, if various routes and modes of transportation are available for individual travelers to choose from, and if travelers are well-informed about options available, then travelers

226 See generally Congressional Budget Office, *Geographic Variation in Health Care Spending*, Feb. 2008, available at http://www.cbo.gov/ftpdocs/89xx/doc8972/02-15-GeogHealth.pdf. See also Baker L., Fisher E., Wennberg J. Variations in Hospital Resource Use For Medicare And Privately Insured Populations in California, Feb. 12, 2008 at http://content.healthaffairs.org/cgi/content/full/hlthaff.27.2.w123/DC1 (evidence that the amount of resources used in the care of chronically ill patients varies widely across hospitals, regardless of the type of insurance coverage).

will make whatever choices best fit their situations. The transportation system should provide a range of choices that fits the existing range of individual needs, but the system should not predetermine some particular pattern of collective choices as the best outcome.

2. *Medical practice and research*

Within that person's unique pathophysiology are elements that medical science is able to understand and/or manipulate therapeutically, to some degree. This scientific knowledge is expressed in terms of elements occurring across a population, abstracted from the unique individuals to whom they apply. But effectively applying that general knowledge to specific individuals very often requires delving into their uniqueness.

How can practitioners and patients apply population-based knowledge to unique individuals in an organized way without being overwhelmed by complexity? And how can clinical researchers and basic scientists systematically test existing knowledge and harvest new knowledge from practitioners' daily encounters with unique patients? The solution to both these problems lies in the tools and standards we use in recording, communicating and processing information.

We have discussed at length how the combinatorial standard for conducting the initial workup and the POMR standard for medical records make it possible to cope with the enormous complexity of medically unique individuals. Here we would reiterate how this happens with the combinatorial standard. A diagnostic or therapeutic problem is defined in terms of sets of clinical findings, based on the medical literature. Then the task is to match the set of findings in the patient with the many sets of findings defined in the knowledge coupling software. The software performs that matching directly. In contrast, the unaided mind resorts to various indirect shortcuts, such as logical inference and probabilities derived from large populations. The difference between these two approaches is like the difference between using an X-ray to view a chest lesion directly, and using a stethoscope to find indirect evidence of what cannot be viewed directly.

Using the more direct, combinatorial approach to match patients against medical knowledge, we constantly encounter individuals who turn out not to match neatly with reported patterns in the medical literature. For example, finding sets on a patient may vary dramatically at different points in the course of a disease, and finding sets frequently suggest numerous diagnostic or therapeutic possibilities, none of which turns out be a good match with the patient. These frequent discrepancies call into question whether accepted "diagnoses" are consistently recognizable, and whether standard treatments should be accepted as standard. This kind of uncertainty in medicine exists elsewhere in biology. Taxonomies established with a tentative and provisional status are then repeatedly applied in a self-reinforcing, circular manner, investing them with an appearance of objective and definable reality that they do not possess.[227]

In medicine, the analogous process is that we use tentative, provisional concepts of diagnosis and treatment to develop algorithms, decision trees, and probability data, which we then apply repeatedly and uncritically. It is as if astronomers theorized about the universe without ever looking through telescopes to test the theories. In medicine, we must build telescopes for seeing beyond current medical "knowledge." This can only be accomplished by using knowledge coupling tools and structured medical records to create a massive, evolving database of patient care. This database would be built on a secure foundation, in two ways:

- The database would be trustworthy because its data inputs would come from practitioners who are continuously held to a high level of performance in executing medical procedures (see part VIII.A.3 below). No longer would there be questions about whether the effects of those procedures reflect variations in the quality of practitioner performance.

- The database would be an extraordinarily rich subject for clinical research, because every item of data could be connected to a structured medical record revealing the original context. That context would be a specific point in the care of a specific problem for a specific individual. The record would reflect the individual's complete history and the practitioner's assessments and planning for each action taken.

With a foundation of carefully executed and rigorously documented processes of care, a database of this kind would open up a deeper view of medical reality than we have ever had before.

As an example, consider the central component of the POMR—the problem list. The list as a whole presents the patient's unique combination of conditions, thereby summarizing the patient's "own peculiar, personal, novel, complicated disease, unknown to medicine" as Tolstoy described it. At the same time, the items on the problem list separate out distinct elements of the patient's personal condition in terms of what is known to medical science. The researcher's

---

227 See Sneath P.H.A and Sokal R., *Numerical Taxonomy: The Principles and Practices of Numerical Classification* (San Francisco: W.H. Freeman & Co., 1973).

scrutiny of any item on the problem list can thus take into account other items on the list,. As described by Dr. Ian Lawson over 35 years ago:

> the POMR system is affecting nosography, the way in which disease and disability are described. ... the interrelationships of problems are as important as the individual problems themselves. Symptoms and problem profiles, rather than summary diagnostic labels, often prove more sensitive in therapeutic management and may eventually lead to a different kind of care organization and epidemiology.[228]

But the advances envisioned by Dr. Lawson have never been fully realized, because the POMR standard of care has never been rigorously enforced, much less enforced in conjunction with the use of knowledge coupling software.

With the ongoing revolution in genomics and proteomics, the myriad resemblances and differences among individual human beings are becoming far more sharply defined at the molecular level. These advances are already making it possible to reconceive existing diagnostic entities, classifications and therapeutic understanding. But to fulfill their potential, these advances require more complete, organized, documented clinical observations in patient care, plus better linkages among these observations and existing knowledge. Were that to occur, there is reason to believe that we would learn how seemingly distinct disease conditions may actually be interrelated, how medical interventions that seem narrowly targeted at a specific gene or molecular pathway may actually disrupt multiple body systems, of how an individual's phenotype may actually be more important than genotype for some diagnostic and therapeutic purposes, and how drugs and other powerful interventions sometimes may be more disruptive and less effective therapeutically than simple improvements in health behaviors. These possibilities are reinforced by evidence that common disease conditions appear linked to many rare genetic variants among individuals rather than to a few common variants across populations.[229]

---

228 Lawson I. Comments on the POMR. In Driggs MF ed. *Problem-Directed and Medical Information Systems*. New York: Inter-Continental Medical Book Corporation, 1974, p. 40. Dr. Lawson goes on to observe: "More to the point, this will also create immediate conflicts with "third party" agents and their prototype definitions of "eligible" illness. Indeed, the sooner their computer experience gets wise to (or gets "blown" by) the realities of multiproblem interrelational analysis and management, the better for us all." See also Graves S. Records as a Tool in Clinical Investigation, in *Applying the Problem-Oriented System*, note 174 above, pp. 272-85, especially its discussion of the concepts of problem list evolution, problem evolution and matching.

229 Heng, H. The Conflict Between Complex Systems and Reductionism, *JAMA* 300;13: 1580-1581 (Oct. 1, 2008). See also Wade N., A Dissenting Voice as the Genome is Sifted to Fight Disease, New York *Times*, Sep. 16, 2008, which states: "the effort to nail down the genetics of most common diseases is not working. ... The common disease/common [genetic] variant idea is

The massive scope and intricacy of our increasing knowledge, and its infinitely variable applicability to individuals, make it increasingly obvious that the minds of highly educated physicians cannot be relied upon to recognize the patterns that define unique individuals and their medical needs. In that environment, we will heed Bacon's warning not to "falsely admire and extol the powers of the human mind," and we will embrace the use of external tools to empower the mind.

Both the mind and external tools use language to reference clinical concepts. Lack of precision and consistency in the use of language has long been recognized as an obstacle to semantic interoperability among disparate health information technologies, particularly electronic health records. Accordingly, major efforts have been underway for many years to develop standardized medical terminology, taxonomies of medical concepts and corresponding coding systems. These efforts, however, valuable as they are, leave unresolved the problem of unstructured clinical judgment by physicians. For example, using standardized terminology to record the results of an initial workup does not assure that the contents of the initial workup will be complete or accurately coupled with medical knowledge. Assuring those goals requires some form of knowledge coupling tools as described above. Standardized terminology and coding is pursued most fruitfully when it is driven by needs that arise in developing knowledge coupling tools and using those tools in medical practice.[230]

Knowledge coupling tools are derived from and linked in detail to an underlying electronic "Knowledge Network," which in turn is derived from and linked to the medical literature. The Knowledge Network is composed of explicitly defined medical entities (findings, disease conditions, medical procedures) and interrelationships among those entities. Standardized terminology and coding of these entities and relationships, when mapped to the Knowledge Network and applied through knowledge coupling software, has far more utility than the same standardized terminology and coding employed in an unstructured manner by physicians. For example:

- Building a module of knowledge coupling software (a "Coupler") for a given medical problem involves defining relationships among numerous medical entities (for example, a disease entity and the finding entities used to diagnose the disease). As the Knowledge Network is built up, it naturally reveals new entity relationships that may not be apparent from reviewing the medical literature (for example, a diagnostic entity may also be a

---

largely wrong. What has happened is that a multitude of rare variants lie at the root of most common diseases ...." See also Moalem, S., Prince J. *Survival of the Sickest: A Medical Maverick Discovers Why We Need Disease.* HarperCollins, 2007.

230 See *Knowledge Coupling*, note 2 above, p. 188.

finding entity in relation to another diagnosis, so that the original finding entities indirectly are related to the second diagnostic entity). When a new Coupler is built for a different medical problem, the existing Knowledge Network is traversed for relevant entities and relationships among them (to continue the example, the indirect relationship between the finding entities and the second diagnostic entity might be relevant to the building of the new Coupler, though not to the first Coupler). Traversing the Knowledge Network may thus reveal connections that medical literature searches would not reveal or reveal only with great difficulty.

• The Knowledge Network content includes not only entity and relationship information but also (1) classifying information that allows entities and relationships to be grouped and retrieved in various ways, and (2) textual explanation of the significance of the entities and relationships. The Knowledge Network thus provides a highly efficient repository of distilled medical knowledge useful for constructing clinical guidance tools—the Couplers.

• Couplers organize information from the Knowledge Network in a problem-oriented manner, that is, in a manner relevant to the specific problem-solving context for which the Coupler is built. The ability to traverse the Knowledge Network for knowledge relevant to the problem context makes it possible to partially automate the process of building Couplers. But this automated element is only the first step. Much thought goes into selecting and editing Knowledge Network content to make it maximally useful in the problem context addressed by the Coupler.

• The Knowledge Network's detailed, organized, interconnected information on medical entities and their properties and interrelationships facilitates use of electronic, problem-oriented medical records with far more consistency, reliability and flexibility than is otherwise possible.[231]

• The volume of medical literature is growing exponentially, much more so than the volume of actionable medical knowledge within the literature. A primary reason is that each article devotes much space to explaining the context and significance of its subject matter, so that related articles consume much space with overlapping explanation. Yet, that explanation does not usually address all of the various medical specialties to which the subject matter is relevant. In contrast, knowledge coupling software and its underlying Knowledge Network enables each piece of actionable knowledge to be expressed concisely and then viewed as needed in the countless medical contexts and specialties to which it may become relevant. Enabling such access to directly relevant knowledge in specific problem solving contexts is far more efficient and effective than ordinary medical literature as a mechanism for storage, retrieval and transmission of medical knowledge.

- Enormous time, money and talent are currently invested in graduate medical education, publication of medical literature, medical libraries, and conferences. All these are mechanisms for transmitting medical knowledge to practitioners using that knowledge. The voltage drop in these transmissions is enormous. Patients have no assurance that the information residing in the minds of their practitioners corresponds to their individual medical needs. In contrast, knowledge coupling tools and the underlying Knowledge Network make it possible to reallocate scarce resources from medical education to medical practice, from futile attempts at teaching medical knowledge to productive *use* of knowledge. And they make it possible to reconceive education itself, based on John Dewey's ideal of knowledge as a "network of interconnections" for exploration.[232]

---

232 See note 294 below.

VIII.
Medical Education and Credentialing as Barriers to Progress

A. Extending the health care reform agenda to medical education and credentialing

1. *A century of stagnation*

Productive use of advanced medical knowledge requires an integrated system of care with a rational division of labor in which all participants see clearly how their roles contribute to solving medical problems. All participants should be able to avail themselves of knowledge that individually they do not possess, practitioners should not be permitted to perform at a level beyond their demonstrated competence, and no group of practitioners should be able to pursue its own interests to the detriment of the larger system of care.

Progress towards a rational division of labor within an external network of knowledge tools is largely absent. Isolated advances are not evolving and coalescing into an integrated system of care. We all are trapped in a non-system, where an elite class of practitioners is permitted to rely on limited personal knowledge and intellect. Graduate medical education and credentialing protect this physician elite from competition that could otherwise reshape medical practice. The health care system has thus been remarkably slow to adapt to the new environment created by modern information technologies. And that environment is still developing. Our culture is still working out the right division of labor between human cognition and external information tools. The subculture of education, however, lags far behind the domains of science and commerce in that development.

Given this state of affairs, and given the need for an integrated system of care, how should medical education and credentialing be reformed? To better understand that question, it is useful to look back a century ago to Abraham Flexner's famous 1910 report on medical education. At that time, many physicians were educated outside of universities. They attended trade schools with low admissions standards, and much of their learning occurred through apprenticeship. Their training did not keep up with scientific advances. Rejecting this model, Flexner advocated the Johns Hopkins, post-graduate model of education, founded in basic science, conducted at universities, and oriented towards research, not practice. As described by Paul Starr, Flexner saw that "a great discrepancy had opened up between medical science and medical education. While science had progressed, education had lagged behind. 'Society reaps at this moment but a small fraction of the advantage which current knowledge has the power to confer.'"[233]

Were Flexner to return today, he would find that current knowledge has the power to confer vastly greater advantage than it did a century ago. But he would not find that society reaps a greater fraction of that advantage. "Between the health care that we have and the care we could have lies not just a gap but a chasm," the Institute of Medicine has found.[234] Failings in medical education and credentialing are a central reason the chasm exists.

These failings are rooted in Flexner's embrace of the university model of formal education. This model was seen as the only way to bring scientific advances to medical practice. Scientific advances were viewed as advances in knowledge, overlooking the advances in intellectual behavior that engendered modern science (as Bacon envisioned). And knowledge was seen as residing in the human mind (Karl Popper's World 2), rather than as objective content existing independently of the mind (World 3) (see the discussion at note 108 above). Flexner thus missed the crucial insight of his contemporary, Whitehead, who saw that civilization advances by lessening dependence on human thought — an insight that Hayek applied to the domain of commerce (see our discussion at notes 103 and 133 above). By missing this point, Flexner helped erect a barrier to quality care in medically underserved communities. The barrier is dependence on highly educated, expensive physicians who do not come from those communities. Affordable training in medicine for local inhabitants must have become more difficult to find after the Flexner reforms. The loss to local communities from this phenomenon is not just reduced access to affordable care. The deeper loss is a decline in quality of care, resulting from cultural disconnect between physician outsiders and local patients. As compared to outsiders, practitioners drawn from the patient population can deliver better care

---

233 Starr P., *The Social Transformation of American Medicine*. New York, Basic Books, 1982. p. 120, quoting Abraham Flexner, *Medical education in the United States and Canada*, Bulletin No. 4, New York, Carnegie Foundation for the Advancement of Teaching, 1910.

234 *Crossing the Quality Chasm*, note 146 above, p. 1.

by reason of their personal relationships with patients and personal knowledge of the community. No medical training can create these connections.[235]

Now, at the centennial of the Flexner report, its basic perspective remains in place. The health care reform legislation does not contemplate fundamental change in medical education and credentialing, and that issue is not even on the agenda for the future. In particular, the concept of the highly educated physician at the top of the hierarchy of practitioners is still accepted as inherent in advanced medical practice.

This point of view ignores what Francis Bacon and modern cognitive psychology have shown about the limits of the mind. It ignores Karl Popper's distinction between World 2 and World 3. It ignores John Dewey's insight that education must be tied to experience, that learning depends upon doing (discussed below). It ignores powerful critiques of credentialing systems based on formal education. It ignores the turning point in medicine's history that modern information technology represents. It ignores the reality that Flexner's approach led practitioners away from using information technology for what should be its core function—combinatorial analysis. And it ignores the experience of graduate medical education—for many, an experience of disillusionment.

2. *The medical school experience*

According to the Institute of Medicine, "many believe that, in general, the current curriculum is overcrowded and relies too much on memorizing facts" and that "the fundamental approach to clinical education has not changed since 1910." Even though the issue is largely absent from the health care reform agenda, many involved in medical education recognize that this stagnation is unacceptable.[236] Consider the following 2003 commentary on Harvard's New Pathway curriculum. After reciting that this reform "reinvigorated the educational experience" and "served as a national model for similar reforms," Dr. Joseph Martin described the sense of futility felt by many:

> But despite all the New Pathway has accomplished, one of its central aims— the true integration of clinical and basic science learning throughout four years of medical school—remains a largely unfulfilled promise.
>
> … There is a pervasive and growing sense—not only at Harvard but around the country—that current approaches are no longer working.

---

235 A further loss to underserved communities is lack of upward mobility for most of the health care workforce, as discussed in below at part VIII.B.2.

236 *Ibid.*, p. 226.

Let me report on some of the observations that have defined this sense of unease with the clinical phase of the student experience.

- Hospital inpatient services are becoming less representative of the full spectrum of illness and patient experience. *Rapid patient turnover limits opportunities for students to develop relationships with patients and follow their progress over time.*

- The increased pace and intensity of the hospital environment makes it less hospitable to the educational needs of students, who are often marginalized as members of inpatient teams. For example, *students rarely take a history or perform a physical exam on patients.*

- Clinical faculty – particularly senior faculty – are less involved in students' education, and a student's contact with a faculty member may be transient.

- *Ambulatory care operates with severe time constraints, compromising the ability of students to learn well in those settings.*

- Evaluation of student performance is highly variable. The lack of direct observation of students by faculty is a major problem in both inpatient and outpatient settings. *The tools used to assess students are not very useful in discerning whether they have achieved core competency.*

- Students receive too little opportunity to appreciate the importance of science as the underpinning of clinical medicine, and to address social, ethical, cultural and professional issues. And finally,

- *The variability in the content and educational rigor of the clinical experience is unacceptable.* Students are often not provided with explicit clinical goals. …

[A] major overarching concern is that *basic science and clinical medicine are not well integrated* across the four year curriculum. Students lack clinical experience in the early years, and basic science is largely ignored in the latter years.[237]

---

237 Martin J. "Outside the Box," *Harvard Medical Alumni Bulletin,* Summer 2003, pp. 38-41, at p. 40 (emphasis added).

This is a remarkable statement. The core purpose of Flexner's reforms was to bring scientific knowledge and rigor to medical practice. A core justification for the enormous time and expense of physician training, and for the legal monopoly and high compensation conferred on physicians, is their scientific training. Presumably that training enables physicians to apply medical science to patient needs with scientific rigor. Yet, one of the leading medical schools in the world here describes itself as failing to provide adequate experience in the elements of clinical medicine, failing to provide good learning conditions in either hospital and ambulatory settings, failing to provide uniformity of content, failing to enforce educational rigor, failing to reliably evaluate students' core competency and failing to integrate basic science and clinical medicine.[238]

Failure to integrate the two is predictable, given what happens in the medical school curriculum.[239] At the beginning, faculties overload students with abstract knowledge—textbook answers to questions they never asked about observations they never made. Learning of this kind is the antithesis of scientific inquiry. Students who undergo this process can easily become doctors who "quote what is in the book and deny what is in the bed." A number of studies, for example, have documented the phenomenon of students who unconsciously "fabricate" findings in patient examinations, perhaps because the findings "are consistent

---

238 The following draws heavily on part III.B of "Opening the Black Box of Clinical Judgment," note 2 above.

239 This failure was anticipated by Dr. William Osler and others at the time of the Flexner Report. They dissented from Flexner's elevation of academic work over clinical experience. See *The Life of Sir William Osler*, note 121 above, Vol. II, p. 292, which quotes Osler as stating: "The ideals would change, and I fear lest the broad open spirit which has characterized the school should narrow, as teacher and student chased each other down the fascinating road of research, forgetful of those whose wider interests to which a great hospital must minister." The history of this dispute is traced in Dr. Michael Lepore's *Death of the Clinician* (Springfield: Charles C. Thomas, 1982). Dr. Lepore quotes a contemporary of Flexner's, Dr. Arthur Dean Bevan, who wrote: "'the medical school cannot be safely left in the hands of the universities alone; something more is needed. Uprooted from the medical profession, uprooted from the community, and transplanted to the scientifically prepared soil of the university campus, the medical school will lack those things which the medical profession and the community alone can give.'" *Ibid.*, p. 30, quoting Bevan, Cooperation in medical education and medical service. *JAMA* 90:15; 1173-1177, Apr. 14, 1928. Others during this period criticized medicine's increasing specialization, which was tied to its academic orientation. A leading cardiologist wrote that he was "opposed to ... journals devoted to the study of specific viscera." He believed that the study of heart disease "lost a great deal of significance" after the journal *Heart* was founded in 1909, "on account of its divorce from the main current of clinical medicine." And Osler's successor at Hopkins criticized the narrowness and "piece worker" aspects of specialization, and its failure to consider the patient as a whole. See Howell J., Reflections on the Past and Future of Primary Care," *Health Affairs*, 29:5; 760-65 (May 2010). See also pages 122-23 of Paul Starr's volume (note 233 above), stating that Flexner himself "became increasingly disenchanted with the rigidity of the educational standards that had become identified with his name."

with their understanding of the disease believed to exist or because they are consistent with the 'classic presentation' of the disease felt to be most likely."[240]

After the beginning curriculum, medical students are thrust into clinical settings with the hope that they will somehow learn to apply their abstract knowledge to real patients effectively while mastering a broad range of manual skills. Yet, absent are the optimal conditions for learning—manageable scope, an individualized program, the opportunity for single-minded attention, careful progression from simple to complex tasks, close feedback. Learning tends to happen on a "sink or swim" basis, with students often left to their own devices, receiving less structure and less organized feedback than in their formal education. The environments in which students are placed do not assure mastery of essential skills. Nor do these environments foster the disciplined behaviors that medical decision making demands. Indeed, the medical school environment violates a basic educational principle stated by John Dewey: "We never educate directly, but indirectly by means of the environment. Whether we permit chance environments to do the work, or whether we design environments for the purpose makes a great difference."[241]

Teaching skills and behaviors is not emphasized in medical education. Rather, its "traditional emphasis is on teaching a *core of knowledge*, much of it focused on the basic mechanisms of disease and pathophysiological principles."[242] But no definable core of knowledge is actually transmitted to or used by practitioners in patient care with any kind of uniformity. Whatever core of knowledge medical schools attempt to teach varies from one institution to another, students do not learn all they are taught, they retain only part of what they do learn, that residue varies with each individual, and some of that residue quickly becomes obsolete. Continuing education courses merely continue this futility. It should thus come as no surprise that continuing education has been found ineffective.[243]

Even if a uniform core of knowledge could be defined and transmitted to students, the students are left with the problem of recalling abstract knowledge

---

240 Friedman M, Connell K, Olthoff A, Sinacore J, Bordage G. Thinking about student thinking: medical student errors in making a diagnosis. *Acad Med.* 1998;73(No. 10/Oct. Supp):S19-S21. Evidence-based medicine promotes a similar phenomenon among practitioners. See Groopman, J., *How Doctors Think*, note 11 above, pp. 138-39 (describing "young physicians who relinquish their own thinking and instead look to classification schemes and algorithms to think for them," and further describing the psychological pressures to refrain from exploring individualized therapies and persist in familiar therapies that are not working).

241 Dewey J. *Democracy and Education: An Introduction to the Philosophy of Education* 1918 (p. 18).

242 *Crossing the Quality Chasm*, note 146 above, p. 210 (emphasis added).

243 Davis D, Thomson M, Oxman A, Haynes B. Changing physician performance: a systematic review of the effect of continuing medical education strategies. *JAMA* 1995; 274:705-705.

presented by a highly specialized faculty and synthesizing it with detailed patient data. A basic assumption of medical education is that the necessary synthesis will somehow spontaneously occur with talented minds. But this synthesis by no means may be assumed. Synthesis depends on the mind's limited capacity to match vast knowledge with detailed data. Moreover, teaching medical knowledge in isolation from patient care is intellectually harmful. Applying the rough generalizations of medical knowledge to the uniqueness of individual patients, and experiencing the imperfect fit between the two, is essential to medical education. This reflects a broader point made by John Dewey: "The most direct blow at the traditional separation of doing and knowing and at the traditional prestige of purely "intellectual" studies, however, has been given by the progress of experimental science. If this progress has demonstrated anything, it is that there is no such thing as genuine knowledge and fruitful understanding except as the offspring of doing."[244]

In this regard, the first two years of medical school resemble the sterile university education that Francis Bacon condemned 400 years ago. The behavior expected of medical students is like the behavior of university students in the late 16th century. They accepted the facts and premises stated by the authority figures who taught them. The approach was not empirical. Logic and formal disputation within this universe of facts and premises prevailed. Ancient authorities were not questioned. Aristotle's authority at Oxford was so great that students were fined five shillings for every point of divergence from his doctrines.[245]

Similarly, medical students are asked to accept the core of knowledge selected and doled out to them by medical school faculties. They are asked to believe that they would be able to retain the endless litany of facts and use them effectively in

244 Dewey J. *Democracy and Education*, note 241 above (p. 321). Louis Menand has further explained Dewey's view: " ... knowledge is a by-product of activity: people do things in the world, and that doing results in learning something that, if deemed useful, gets carried along into the next activity. In the traditional method of education in which the things considered worth knowing are handed down from teacher to pupil as disembodied information, knowledge is cut off from the activity in which it has its meaning, and becomes a false abstraction. One of the consequences (besides boredom) is that an invidious distinction between knowing and doing—a distinction Dewey thought socially pernicious as well as philosophically erroneous—gets reinforced." *The Metaphysical Club* (New York: Farrar, Straus and Giroux, 2001), p. 322. See also Thomas Sowell's critique of purely intellectual studies in *Knowledge and Decisions*, note 129 above, at pp. 9-10 (discussing the possibility that as people acquire "more schooling, ... their standards for 'knowing' decline while the area of their secondhand and tenuous knowledge expands"), p. 41 (discussing "direct knowledge of the particulars of time and place, as distinguished from the secondhand generalities known as 'expertise,'" p. 150 (distinguishing between socially effective knowledge or feedback and mere articulation of information), pp. 214-218 (the limitations of articulated knowledge), pp. 334-38 (limits of the intellectual process).

245 Gaukroger, note 112 above, p. 39 n. 10.

the care of patients in the years ahead. And they are not placed in environments of scientific inquiry. On the contrary:

> ... health care settings are among the most hierarchical in American society. In these settings, students, residents, nurses, pharmacists, and other health care workers are often intimidated by physicians and reluctant to question decisions or offer alternative views. These are the frameworks in which student values, attitudes and behaviors are shaped. The science content-packed curriculum reinforces these frameworks by its emphasis on the acquired knowledge and primacy of the individual physician and his/her judgment.[246]

In assuming that students must be indoctrinated with received knowledge as preparation for real patient care, medical schools trap student minds in what Tolstoy called "the snare of preparation." Like a drug, such education has toxicity as well as benefit. One of its toxic effects is to reinforce a basic human need to deny uncertainty. Dr. Jay Katz has described "how readily any awareness of uncertainty succumbs to venerable authority and orthodoxy. These powerful defenses against awareness of uncertainty continue to rule professional practices."[247] Sociologist Robert Weaver has further described findings in the literature on this phenomenon:

> A major task undertaken during medical training is learning to manage the uncertainty associated with medicine and medical education. For instance, medical students learn the disadvantages of "doubting too much" and displaying these doubts to peers, superiors, and patients. Instead, they often develop a misleading sense of certitude or come to don a "cloak of competence" to help them manage the impressions of others and, ultimately, the image they have of themselves. Confidence and belief in what one is doing is a central component of the "clinical mentality" as Friedson describes it. Doubts about the ambiguities of "unusual" cases, even when acknowledged by the practitioner, are often "silenced" or otherwise not shared with the patient.[248]

---

246 *Unmet Needs: Teaching Physicians to Provide Safe Patient Care.* Report of the Lucian Leape Institute Roundtable on Reforming Medical Education (2010), pp. 9-10, available at http://www.npsf.org/LLI-Unmet-Needs-Report. This report goes on to describe the "disruptive and abusive behavior" by teaching staff to which medical students are sometimes subjected in their clinical training (pp. 10-120).

247 Katz J. *The silent world of doctor and patient.* New York: Free Press - Macmillan, 1984. p. 179.

248 Weaver R. Clinical uncertainty, responsibility and change in medical practice: a socio-

Medical students emerge from this process with insufficient sensitivity to patient uniqueness and the fallibility of medical knowledge.

Medical education must be reformed to produce practitioners who are resistant to the generalizations and misconceptions of their teachers, who are equipped with scientific habits of rigor and independent inquiry. For this to happen, the only workable mode of education is careful engagement of students in patient care itself. Students must *use* knowledge rather than learn it in the abstract. They must rely on information tools to access all relevant knowledge rather than erudition to access limited personal knowledge. If the worlds of action and knowledge do not connect easily and securely in this way, then good students become cynical and distrustful rather than fully engaged.[249]

The premises of medical education, the legal authority it confers to act upon unaided judgment, and the financial and social rewards for doing so, tend to reinforce basic traits of human nature—faith in one's own cognitions and insensitivity to one's own ignorance—traits that undermine scientific rigor in medical practice. Francis Bacon long ago observed the tension between science and the mind's normal mode of operation: "The human understanding, when any proposition has been once laid down, . . . forces everything else to add fresh support and confirmation . . . rather than sacrifice the authority of its first conclusions."[250] Although medical school faculties, students and practitioners try to overcome this basic human trait, their attempts inevitably fall short of what properly designed software tools and medical records can achieve. With the rigorous combinatorial analysis that those devices facilitate in a disciplined environment, the realities of individual patients continually generate rapid, organized, cumulative feedback on the hypotheses of practitioners and the generalizations of medical knowledge. Such feedback represents a superior medical education for all practitioners. "By contrast, our present educational premises and overuse of statistical thinking tend to confirm and buttress past notions, right or wrong. Above all they stifle progress toward expecting and dealing honestly with the ultimate uniqueness of each patient."[251]

---

logical response to Weed's knowledge coupling innovation. (citations omitted) Weaver, R. R. (2002). "Resistance to computer innovation: knowledge coupling in clinical practice." *SIGCAS Comput. Soc.* 32(1): 16-21 p. 18).

249 Weed LL. A Touchstone for Medical Education. *Harvard Medical Alumni Bulletin.* 1974 (Nov./Dec.): 13-18. See also Geoffrey Norman's discussion of the psychological advantages of using patient problems to teach clinical concepts, at pp. 282-83 of "Problem-solving skills, solving problems and problem-based learning," note 96 above. Dr. Norman wrote about the traditional paradigm of *learning* knowledge, but his discussion applies even more when we seek to *access* and *apply* knowledge rather than learn it.

250 Bacon F. *Novum Organum* (1620), note 1 above, Aphorism No. 46.

251 Weed CC. Philosophy, interpretation and use of problem-knowledge couplers, note 2

3. *Changing medical education from a knowledge-based to a skills-based approach*

At a time when medical knowledge far exceeds the capacity of the human mind to learn it, when knowledge is more accessible than ever before, when medical knowledge can be coupled with patient data using external tools, it no longer makes sense to conceive medical education in terms of learning knowledge. Nor does it make sense to license practitioners based on their undergoing didactic education and passing board examinations on the limited knowledge they temporarily learn. Both students and practitioners need to access and apply knowledge, not learn it. What needs to be learned is a core of behavior, not a core of knowledge. The required behaviors are defined by the system's standards of care. In general terms, the required behaviors have four dimensions: thoroughness (does the practitioner consistently perform all required tasks); reliability (does the practitioner perform each task with the required level of skill); analytic sense (can the practitioner provide a rational basis for each action taken); and efficiency (does the practitioner complete required tasks with sufficient speed). These four dimensions should be applied to each of the four basic phases of medical action discussed in part VI: the data base, problem list, initial plans and progress notes.[252] Defining and enforcing a core of behavior in these terms is greatly facilitated when electronic records are designed in accordance with the POMR standard.

The futility of learning a core of knowledge becomes even more obvious when one considers that users of medical knowledge include not just physicians but other practitioners, their patients, and consumers who are not relying on practitioners. All need to be able to draw upon comprehensive, objective knowledge—not limited, subjective, personal knowledge (recall the discussion of Karl Popper's World 2 and World 3 at note 108 above).

Anyone who accesses and applies medical knowledge will, of course, learn much in the process. But such individual learning should be a by-product of the activity, not its goal. Learning by individuals is idiosyncratic and subject

above, p. 8. For further discussion of the role of medical records in education, written before development of knowledge coupling software, see *Medical Records, Medical Education and Patient Care* (note 2 above), "A Touchstone for Medical Education (note 249), and Part Three of *The Problem-Oriented System* (note 171). See also Groopman, J., *How Doctors Think*, note 11 above, p. 126 ("In medical school, and later during residency training, the emphasis is on learning the typical picture of a certain disorder, whether it is a peptic ulcer or a kidney stone. Seemingly unusual or atypical presentations often get short shrift.").

252 For further discussion, see Schacher S., Weed, LL. "The New Curriculum," in *The Problem-Oriented System*, note 171 above, pp. 95-104.

to rapid obsolescence. Even if there were some useful core of knowledge that could be uniformly learned by practitioners and never go out-of-date, that core of knowledge is not enough for any individual patient. The varying knowledge relevant to each patient will rarely correspond to the limited knowledge that happens to reside in the minds of the practitioners the patient happens to encounter. Moreover, the patient has no assurance that practitioners will act objectively in coupling knowledge with patient data. To be trustworthy and transparent, the storage, retrieval and initial processing of medical knowledge must be carried out through an external system or network that practitioners and patients jointly access. Cognitive inputs to patient care generated in this manner are subject to definition, control and continuous improvement.

Beyond applying medical knowledge, practitioners must skillfully perform medical procedures. Neither data collection nor execution of decisions is trustworthy unless skill is assured in performance of the procedures involved. Similarly, outcome studies of diagnostic and therapeutic procedures are not meaningful unless skillful performance is assured (unfavorable outcomes could be attributable to lack of skill rather than lack of efficacy). In short, practitioner inputs to performance of medical procedures must be defined and controlled no less than cognitive inputs to decision making.

How is this to be done? A model exists in another professional arena where public safety is at stake: licensing of commercial airline pilots. James Fallows has described this approach to credentialing:

> The pilot-licensing system was built on the premise that competence was divisible. People can be good at one thing without being good at others, and they should be allowed to do only what they have mastered. As opposed to receiving a blanket license, the way members of other professions do, pilots must work their way up through four certificate levels, from student to air-transport pilot, and be specifically qualified on each kind of aircraft they want to fly. What's more, a pilot must demonstrate at regular intervals that he is still competent. To keep his license a pilot must take a review flight with an instructor every two years, and the pilots for commercial airlines must pass a battery of requalification tests every six months.[253]

---

253 James Fallows, "The Case Against Credentialism," *The Atlantic Monthly* (Dec 1985), pp. 65-66, available at http://jamesfallows.theatlantic.com/archives/1985/12/the_case_against_credentialism.php. Contrary to what Fallows' title might suggest and contrary to Milton Friedman's view (discussed at note 269 below), this book does not oppose credentialing but instead advocates *better* credentialing, based not on didactic education but on demonstrated competence in discrete skills.

This regulatory scheme differs from traditional, knowledge-based credentialing by recognizing some fundamental principles. The common element underlying these principles is that inputs by the professional are defined, controlled and transparent:

- *Actual demonstration of skillful, competent performance, not success in formal, didactic education, must be the basis for licensure.* Knowledge-based education demonstrates preparation, not actual performance.

- *Unlike knowledge, skillful performance can only be learned firsthand, by doing.* Secondhand learning by reading or listening or observing is never enough to acquire competence in the hands-on skills needed from expert practitioners.

- *License to practice should be defined and conferred only for discrete skills.* Stated differently, demonstrated competence in one skill should not confer a license to practice other skills. Thus, for example, inputs by commercial pilots are tightly defined; they are "specifically qualified on each kind of aircraft they want to fly," not to fly aircraft in general.

- *The minimum standard for licensure must be set at a high level.* Thus, individuals "should be allowed to do only what they have mastered," as with airline pilot licensing. Activities where safety is at stake differ from other activities in this regard. In many economic contexts, consumers want the opportunity for trade-offs between cost and quality, which means producers should have the freedom to offer those trade-offs. But in activities like airline travel and health care, those trade-offs are unacceptable where safety is compromised, which means that inputs by producers must be tightly controlled (as further discussed in part VIII.B.1).

- *Licensure should be temporary.* A degree or license received at the beginning of a career should not confer a permanent entitlement to practice. The only way to control the quality of inputs from practitioners over time is periodic scrutiny of inputs.

These principles from aviation are not just an optional alternative to traditional credentialing in medicine; they are the only viable approach. Some might view this approach as less rigorous than traditional credentialing because it is shorter and less costly, but in fact this approach is *more* rigorous.

Out of necessity, physician training has adapted somewhat to the principles just described, but in an *ad hoc*, muddled, incomplete way. Thus, medical school curricula include both didactic education and learning by doing (apprenticeship), but the two are not well integrated, and both are ineffective. The didactic portion is not just futile but harmful: it separates knowledge from practice while demanding a Sisyphean effort to master vast medical knowledge. This dissipates students' limited time and energy, which would be more productively invested in the apprenticeship portion of medical school, where basic clinical skills should be mastered. Unfortunately, the apprenticeship portion does not offer an adequate opportunity to develop mastery of clinical skills, as described by Dr. Martin above, because rotations from one service to another are too short, superficial and unstructured. As a result, medical school graduates often enter internship and residency without the expected competence in basic skills.

These deficiencies in medical school would be of less concern if subsequent training were adequate, but it is not. Internship and residency programs do not assure development of high levels of personal skill. Nor do they offer new physicians the experience of working within disciplined systems of teamwork and quality control. On the contrary:

> Care is given by a variety of specialists and disciplines working closely under stressful conditions, yet training of the various "tribes" occurs in isolation that reinforces individual cultures and norms. Care is given by "teams," yet classic notions and skills associated with high performance teamwork are never taught to health care professionals. Dangerous, risky procedures are performed by novices or experienced clinicians learning new approaches on actual patients under conditions of, at best, implied consent. The introduction of new complex medical devices into actual care, and the exposure of new employees and trainees to existing medical devices occurs with little or no effective systematic training in the operation and trouble-shooting of these devices. Practitioners' exposure to the range of possible classic events, problems, diseases, crises, and surprises occurs ad hoc, as a by-product of the apprenticeship training model. Hence, the level of experience and competence varies widely among those who have completed training or the first cycles of independent, certified practice.[254]

---

254 Stephen D. Small, Thoughts on Patient Safety Education and the Role of Simulation, *Virtual Mentor*. March 2004, Volume 6, Number 3, http://virtualmentor.ama-assn.org/2004/03/medu1-0403.html.

Medical training thus immerses new physicians in environments of undefined, uncontrolled inputs. This form of training perpetuates a "system that predictably produces the current annual epidemic of medical injuries."[255]

The ordeal endured by new physicians culminates in board certification exams—a reversion to the didactic model of education. With its premise that the human mind can be relied upon to learn and apply medical knowledge, with its acceptance of board certification as the gold standard of credentialing, the didactic model of education embodies medicine's culture of denial.

The opportunity to overcome the failings of knowledge-based education and credentialing is greater now than it has ever been. Information technology can now radically reduce the burden on practitioners of learning medical knowledge. Simulation technologies now permit students to develop some manual skills to a relatively high level before applying their skills to real patients. Teamwork simulation techniques are now known to improve performance of teams in complex, high-stress situations. Indeed, health care lags behind other sectors (for example, the military, the nuclear power industry, commercial aviation and aerospace) in using simulation to teach individual skills and improve team performance.[256]

A skills-based approach to education and credentialing has enormous potential to reduce the time and expense of becoming qualified to deliver care. Rather than spending many years in a futile attempt to master medical knowledge, practitioners could master specific skills in much less time. Regina Herzlinger has described an example suggesting the potential of this approach. The Shouldice Hospital in Toronto specializes in abdominal hernia surgery. The hospital's surgeons perform that procedure alone, averaging six hundred operations per year per surgeon, about 20 times as many as the average general surgeon. Rather than becoming bored, "the Shouldice surgeons view hernia operations as a continual challenge, and like fine craftspeople, they take great pleasure in performing them consistently and reliably."[257] The surgical approach they

---

255 *Ibid.*

256 Halamek L. Simulation-Based Training: Opportunities for the Acquisition of Unique Skills. *Virtual Mentor,* 8:2; 84-87 (Feb. 2006). See also Health Research and Educational Trust, *Resources on Simulation-Based Medical Training,* available at http://www.hret.org/hret/programs/content/simbiblio.pdf, For opposing views on the cost-effectiveness of simulation (Sep. 2006), see Gaba D, What Does Simulation Add to Teamwork Training, http://www.webmm.ahrq.gov/perspective.aspx?perspectiveID=20; Pratt S. Sachs D., Team Training: Classroom Training vs. High-Fidelity Simulation,   http://www.webmm.ahrq.gov/perspective.aspx?perspectiveID=21.

257 Herzlinger, R. *Market-Driven Health Care* (Perseus Books, 1997), pp. 159-63. Professor Herzlinger discusses the Shouldice Hospital in the context of advocating the "focused factory" model of manufacturing for health care. The focused factory model is successful at improving execution inputs for isolated procedures such as abdominal hernia surgery, but a total system of care cannot be so narrow. Practitioners must care for patients as they are, and patient needs are

employ is less invasive and more painstaking than the conventional approach. Learning the nuances and complications that each case potentially presents, these surgeons acquire deep expertise not reflected by their limited formal credentials. When Dr. Atul Gawande observed the Shouldice surgical teams, he concluded, "None of the three surgeons I watched ... would even have been in a position to conduct their own procedures in a typical American hospital, for none had completed general surgery training. ... Yet after apprenticing for a year or so they were the best hernia surgeons in the world."[258]

In aviation, apprenticeship is the core of pilot credentialing. Above we described pilot credentialing in terms of five principles that are no less applicable to medical practitioners. It is no coincidence that the physician who pioneered use of knowledge coupling software with the electronic POMR, Dr. Ken Bartholomew, is a licensed, instrument-rated pilot.[259] In his chapter on practicing medicine with knowledge coupling software and the POMR, Dr. Bartholomew writes, "I continuously see parallels in aviation safety and medicine." He goes on to quote Gerard Bruggink, a retired National Transportation Safety Board expert, who describes professional expertise as a matter not of learning but of character:

> Aviation character is the triumph of humility and common sense over arrogance and overconfidence. ... character governs the quality with which we apply our skills and knowledge to the task at hand. Character generates the mysterious force that often holds things together when aviation's grand design comes apart at the seams. ... Although the most spectacular test of character lies in the handling of a rare emergency, its unremitting test is the monotony of routine operations. It takes more

broad, not focused. In particular, a total health care system must avoid the trap of conferring authority on focused specialists to decide on the need for their own services. This is a recipe for overutilization and fragmented care in a fee-for-service system. In contrast, a fee-for-service system might become highly cost-effective and productive of the highest quality care, if some practitioners focused on expert, efficient execution of discrete medical procedures with no authority to recommend those procedure, while other practitioners focused on helping patients navigate the system to decide what procedures are needed, with those practitioners having no authority to execute the chosen procedures.

258 Gawande A. No Mistake. *The New Yorker* 1998 March 30; p. 111-116. As to the question of whether the best medical care requires fully trained doctors, see part VIII.B.2 below.

259 Dr. Bartholomew has flown-accident-free for over 30 years. He voluntarily flies with an instructor, more often than required by FAA regulations, to review and refresh his skills (which on one occasion enabled him to survive an engine explosion in mid-flight and a "deadstick" landing on a narrow country road). His experience of the need to continuously maintain and improve his skills, as distinguished from relying on his education, made him especially receptive to adopting new tools and standards for his medical practice in 1986 when he first learned about knowledge coupling software. (Personal communication with Dr. Bartholomew.)

than certifiable skills and knowledge to tip the scales in favor of safety when invitations to complacency abound.[260]

Finding these words precisely applicable to medicine, and citing examples of egregious medical errors, Dr. Bartholomew is telling us that every day medicine's grand design comes apart at the seams. Our test of character is to create a new design, to radically reform education and credentialing, to teach and enforce new standards of care. "Let us then use the tools of our age." Dr. Bartholomew writes, "to meet the unremitting test of monotony ... so that a routine case does not become an emergency. Let us begin to use tools ... to give the type of care that we imply by our words and actions we are capable of giving."

B. Marketplace implications of skills-based credentialing

1. Professional autonomy and regulation of practitioners

Traditionally, professional autonomy has been highly valued in the marketplace for health professional services.[261] But the approach to credentialing just described is incompatible with professional autonomy. Airline pilots, for example, do not decide when and where to fly, and they must follow guidance from detailed checklists and procedures, cockpit instruments, and the air traffic control system.

In medicine, credentialing of individual practitioners similarly should not confer authority to depart from procedural guidance, nor authority to decide whether a medical procedure is necessary and appropriate for an individual patient. Rather, credentialing should confer authority only to execute medical decisions within a defined, controlled, integrated system of care. Failure to recognize this principle leads to provider-induced demand for unnecessary and inappropriate services.

---

260 See pp. 247-48 of *Knowledge Coupling*, note 2 above.

261 Autonomy is a goal of not just the medical profession but the professions generally, including university professors. "For professions, unlike other types of occupations, are self-regulating," as Louis Menand has written. "Professions are democratic in the sense that they are open to anyone with talent, but they are guilds in the sense that they protect their members from market forces with which all nonprofessionals have to cope. ... Professionalization is a system of market control." Menand goes on to describe the professionalization of the university, which was "designed to make academic work self-regulating" through such practices as PhD credentialing, publication in peer-reviewed journals as a requirement for advancement, and academic freedom. "Academic freedom is a freedom specifically designed for academics; it can be enjoyed only by people already admitted in the club. ... Academic freedom for a professor is, therefore, actually or potentially, a restriction on everyone who is not a professor." Menand L. *The Metaphysical Club*, note 244 above, pp. 414-15. Having occurred by the time of the Flexner report, this professionalization of the university apparently contributed to the idealization of professional

In the current marketplace, professional autonomy extends not just to decision making but to execution of decisions. That is, autonomous physicians are free to perform at varying levels of proficiency. High standards are not enforced. Although peer review mechanisms and malpractice litigation purport to enforce some standards of performance, those standards are not well defined, and are not set at a high level. Moreover, the marketplace does not consistently reward high standards: patients are not well positioned to assess quality, reimbursement from third party payers is poorly linked with quality of performance, and malpractice litigation is ineffective at distinguishing between high and low quality.

In many economic contexts, it is productive for consumers to be able to choose among a wide range of trade-offs between quality and cost. But this is rarely the case in medicine. In that market, demand for less-than-high-quality performance is minimal, because the usual trade-offs between cost and quality are absent. Several reasons are apparent. Substandard performance can easily cause enormous medical and economic harm; cost and quality often do not correlate; the quality of performance and risk of harm are difficult to judge for consumers and third party payers alike. Consider, for example, a carelessly performed physical examination resulting in a missed or delayed diagnosis of a serious condition that might have been easily treated if detected early. Few patients would bargain with that risk for low cost. Similarly, third party payers could face costs from one such case that outweigh savings obtained by cutting corners in performing physical exams in hundreds of other cases (a point of view that private and public payers are just beginning to recognize, as evidenced by recent announcements that provider reimbursement will be denied for costs resulting from egregious errors[262]). Because of these factors, consumers and third party payers alike have little to gain and much to lose by tolerating less than optimal performance.

In short, standards of performance need to be established and enforced at a high level and then continuously improved as advances in procedures and techniques are developed. Corresponding reimbursement policies need to be applied. Thus enforcing high standards creates an evolutionary process of selecting for performance improvement, so that deficiencies are eliminated and improvements reproduced systematically.

---

autonomy and exclusivity in medicine. (The Flexner report resulted in the closure of numerous medical schools and the requirement for post-graduate medical education as a credential for admission to practice.)

262 See Mantone, J., "Insurers: Hospitals Should Pay For Mistakes, The Wall Street Journal Health Blog," Jan. 15, 2008, available at http://blogs.wsj.com/health/2008/01/15/insurers-hospitals-should-pay-for-mistakes.

All of this depends on a basic cultural change in medicine. Needed is a shift from the ideal of professional autonomy to a standard of clearly defining and rigorously controlling provider inputs to care. To reiterate the words of William Blake: "Art and Science cannot exist but in minutely organized Particulars." This concept explains the power of patient safety advances conceived by leaders such as Don Berwick[263], Lucian Leape[264] and Peter Pronovost.[265] But these advances are not enough. And they will not be generalized and maintained as long as we continue with the system's current foundation, the existing premises and tools.

The patient safety movement originally focused on decision execution. Increasingly, decision making itself has come to be recognized as a patient safety issue. But this recognition is incomplete. Missing is a broader recognition of the essential unity of the problem and the solution, for both decision making and execution. In both arenas, as this book has described, the problem is undefined and uncontrolled inputs by practitioners. The solution is defining practitioner inputs not according to provider habits, or third party dictates, or medical "knowledge." Both patients and practitioners need to function within a tightly defined system of care. The system should enable them to elicit the information needed for individualized problem solving. In situations where established knowledge provides clear solutions to patient problems, no real decision making is needed. In situations of genuine uncertainty, the system should identify alternative possible solutions, with the pros and cons of each, as a basis for decision making by the patient.

What patients then need from providers is reliable and cost-effective execution. Providers (individual practitioners and the institutions where they work) should be able to compete to satisfy this demand. The forces of competition, if permitted to operate, would increasingly reward practitioners who perform as experts within systems that tightly define and control execution inputs. But none of this can happen transforming education and credentialing, without shifting knowledge from minds to tools, without enforcing a core of behavior

2. Transforming the hierarchy of practitioners

This gap between scientific evidence about what works best and the care patients receive calls into question the fundamental basis of the modern physician's authority.

Michael L. Millenson[266]

---

263 See www.ihi.org.

264 See note 123 above.

265 See note 41 above.

266 Millenson M. *Demanding Medical Excellence: Doctors and Accountability in the Information*

Doctors know that medical information systems are inadequate, but unpressured by the current system and a lack of competition, they make excuses for the system and themselves.

Paul A. London[267]

Graduate medical education does not instill the behaviors required to compete on the basis of high quality inputs to care. Non-physician practitioners may prove to be better candidates than physicians to function in a system designed for external information tools, informed decisions, reliable execution and genuine accountability. A system of that kind requires a new division of labor. Yet, changing the division of labor encounters legal barriers to medical practice by non-physician practitioners and further barriers to corporate involvement in practice. Entrepreneurial providers, third party payers and consumer groups are likely to recognize a common interest in removing these legal barriers. Together they would have the political power to do so by overcoming the professional sovereignty of physicians.[268]

Many observers (most prominently Milton Friedman) have argued that occupational licensure in general, and medical licensure in particular,

---

Age (Chicago: University of Chicago Press, 1997), p. 121.

267 London P. *The Competition Solution* (Washington, AEI Press, 2004), p. 193. Authored by an economist and political scientist who served as a deputy undersecretary of commerce for economics and statistics during the Clinton administration, this book attributes the economic dynamism of the 1990's to policy decisions in preceding decades that increased competition in many economic sectors, "despite the strenuous efforts by powerful business and labor interests to limit it. ... The 'special interests' threatened and begged, but they lost, and the country prospered as a result. ... Expanding our prosperity will depend more on future efforts to expand competition in areas like health care and education, which are holding the economy back today, than on tax arrangements and changes in interest rates, which do little to make poorly performing industries more dynamic and successful" (pp. 4-5).

268 See Paul Starr's *The Social Transformation of American Medicine*, note 233 above, discussing the "influence of professional sovereignty on the division of labor in American medicine" (p. 225). Starr describes how that influence advanced the medical profession's economic interests at the expense of other practitioners: "Among physicians, the division of labor was only loosely regulated, but between physicians and other occupations, it was hierarchical and rigid. *The possibilities of moving from nurse or technologist to physician were negligible; experience at one level did not count towards qualification on the next*" (emphasis added). Starr goes on to argue that the medical profession's monopoly prevented corporate enterprises from seeking greater flexibility in the use of practitioners. Corporations "might have tried to substitute the cheaper labor of ancillary workers for physicians in many areas that physicians insisted on retaining. ... The [corporate] firm might also have subjected doctors to more hierarchical control: The physician with limited graduate training might not have been free, for example, to do whatever procedures he considered himself competent to perform. As in other industries, the management of the enterprise might have sought to take away from the workers control over the division of labor, which physicians retained through the system of professional sovereignty." *Ibid.*

restrict competition for the benefit of the regulated professions without commensurate benefit to the public.[269] Indeed, lobbying pressure for licensure statutes comes from occupational groups, not from victims of unregulated labor markets. Medical licensure is especially restrictive because it erects not only a legal barrier to competition but also a high economic barrier—graduate medical education, which is so expensive, time-consuming and difficult to enter that few people can even consider becoming a physician. The resulting monopoly means that physicians spend much of their time providing services that less expensive practitioners could perform. This state of affairs, Friedman emphasizes, not only hinders price competition but also retards innovation in delivery of care:

> There are many different routes to knowledge and learning and the effect
> of restricting the practice of what is called medicine and defining it as we
> tend to do to a particular group, who in the main have to conform to the
> prevailing orthodoxy, is certain to reduce the amount of experimentation
> and hence reduce the rate of growth of knowledge in the area. What is
> true for the content of medicine is also true for its organization …[270]

Friedman concludes that licensure should be eliminated as a requirement for medical practice. He argues that licensure does not assure quality, that the public finds other ways to assess the quality of practitioners, and that a free market would develop better quality assurance than that provided by the current regulated marketplace for health professional services.

Rather than eliminating medical licensure as Friedman suggests, a better alternative is to change medical licensure from a knowledge-based to a skills-based approach. To reiterate, this would require medical practitioners of all kinds to demonstrate periodically skillful performance of discrete skills at a high

269 Friedman M., Kuznets, S. *Income from Independent Professional Practice, 1929-1936* (National Bureau of Economic Research, 1954) (originally published in 1939), available at http://www.nber.org/books/frie54-1; Friedman, M. *Capitalism and Freedom* (Chicago: University of Chicago Press, 1962), pp. 137-60; Svorny S., *Medical Licensing: An Obstacle to Affordable, Quality Care*, Cato Institute Policy Analysis No. 621, Sep. 17, 2008, available at http://www.cato.org/pubs/pas/pa-621.pdf; Kling A, Cannon M., *Does the Doctor Need a Boss?*, Cato Institute Briefing Paper No. 111, Jan. 13, 2009, available at http://www.cato.org/pubs/bp/bp111.pdf; Kleiner M. "Occupational Licensure and the Internet: Issues for Policy Makers," (2002), at http://www.ftc.gov/opp/ecommerce/anticompetitive/panel/kleiner.pdf; Fallows, "The Case Against Credentialism," note 253 above; Gross S., *Of Foxes and Hen Houses: Licensing and the Health Professions*, (Westport, CT: Quorum Books, 1984); Shimberg B, Roederer D. *Occupational Licensing: Questions a Legislator Should Ask* (Lexington, KY, Council on Licensure, Enforcement and Regulation, 2d ed 1994); Collins, R. *The Credential Society: An Historical Sociology of Education and Stratification* (Academic Press, 1979).

270 Friedman, M. *Capitalism and Freedom*, p. 157.

level of quality. Practitioners would rely not on limited personal knowledge, but rather on the infrastructure provided by knowledge coupling tools, to access the knowledge needed for patient care. Credentialing would be based on performance, not training. Quality and patient safety would be better protected, economic barriers to practice would be reduced, and innovation would increase, relative to the current marketplace for health professional services.[271]

Medical specialization already represents a crude form of this approach. Both market and regulatory forces restrict entry to practice in advanced medical specialties, and specialists often then subspecialize further in specific procedures. Reform along these lines can be developed to some extent by health care institutions even within the framework of current state medical practice acts. Provider institutions and third party payers can develop and administer skills-based credentialing for employment of health care professionals, within systems for medical decision making informed by information tools as we have described. Legislative changes would become necessary to the extent that such an environment would enable non-physician practitioners to perform services currently reserved by law to physicians.

Traditional physicians could not compete for patients against non-physician practitioners who function within a tightly defined and rigorous system of care. Such a system would give rise to a free market in high quality professional health services (the market in lesser quality services would naturally contract to areas where consumers can safely trade off cost and quality). Anyone who regularly demonstrated proficiency in a specific medical procedure could be credentialed to perform that procedure, without regard to educational attainment. Training to achieve this proficiency would be far more focused and rigorous than at present. This focused training itself should do much to reduce the high level of execution errors that now occur.

Arbitrary occupational categories like "physician" and "nurse" would disappear. Language would change its meaning. No longer would we define "medical practice" as that which is done by credentialed physicians. Medical practice would instead be defined in terms of providing specific expertise as needed to execute decisions made by patients/consumers. Medical practice in this sense would encompass a multitude of functions, including functions now performed by those labeled as surgeons, internists, nurses, dentists, radiologists, osteopaths, chiropractors, physical therapists, psychiatrists, clinical psychologists, and many others. Most of these categories would subdivide into many roles, each defined by expertise in discrete caregiving functions. All of these practitioners

---

271 See "Physicians of the Future," note 51 above, and part VI of "Reengineering Medicine," note 38 above, for further discussion of these issues.

would function within a rigorously ordered and transparent system of care. None of these practitioners would have the unilateral authority to define the need for their own services. Moreover, support personnel who do not themselves render care to patients would form part of the system of care supporting patients and practitioners.[272]

Collectively, these various occupational roles would call upon the full range of human abilities and acquired expertise. Those with natural interpersonal skills or manual dexterity would thrive in roles where a free market would reward those abilities, without the barrier of arbitrary educational requirements. At the same time, no one would be expected or permitted to perform in roles beyond his or her personal capacity. Each practitioner who performs at a high level while providing the emotional support that patients need from healers would in a very real sense be a physician.[273] In contrast, the current restricted market for health professional services permits physicians to perform a wide range of functions, both within and outside their capacity to perform well, including complex and risky interventions that are better not done at all if not done well.

Little accountability exists for poor performance of medical procedures. Creating accountability requires changing the hierarchy of practitioners. Medicine tolerates defective behaviors and the defective services those behaviors produce at the top of the hierarchy. Dr. Peter Pronovost has confronted this reality in his famous studies of a routine hospital procedure—central line insertions. The procedure risks fatal infection of the bloodstream every time it is performed. "This infection is common, costly, and is associated with the death of 31,000 patients annually in the United States, yet it can be accurately

---

272 See Dr. Ken Bartholomew's description of how introducing the electronic POMR in his office enabled a medical records technician, Zelda Gebhard, to change from being typist in a cubicle to "a real partner in patient care." The POMR "made her think critically about what she is doing, what we are doing, and why we are doing it. With the computerized [POMR], she needed to know what was going on in order to know where a particular note or a particular lab test should be entered. ... Now, it is very easy to think critically about the performance of *locum tenens* physicians as she sees the neatness or sloppiness of their thought processes, whatever may be the case. ... Now, when other physicians work for me, and they make a diagnosis such as strep pharyngitis without having done a streptazyme test or throat culture, [she] brings this to my attention by asking if this should be listed as strep pharyngitis, pharyngitis or simply sore throat. I can see her growing ability to analyze the problem and to apply the rules of clinical evidence to support diagnostic accuracy. It makes me wonder if medical schools have failed overall in teaching doctors to think critically and scientifically about these questions." Bartholomew, note 64 above, pp. 260-61.

273 See "Physicians of the Future," note 51 above, and Bendapudi N. et al. Patient Perspectives on Ideal Physician Behaviors. 2006. *Mayo Clinic Proceedings*, 81(3): 338-344 (based on a patient survey, seven qualities define the ideal physician: confident, empathetic, humane, personal, forthright, respectful, and thorough).

measured and largely prevented [with] a checklist of prevention practices, strict measurement of infection rates, and tools to improve culture and team work among physicians, nurses, and administrators," Dr. Pronovost writes. As part of his studies, Dr. Pronovost asked nurses in participating hospitals, "'if a new nurse in your hospital saw a senior physician placing a catheter but not complying with the checklist, would the nurse speak up and would the physician comply?'" Here is what he found:

> The answer is almost always, 'there is no way the nurse would speak up.' Doubly disturbing, physicians and nurses uniformly agree patients should receive the checklist items. What other industry would accept a routine safety violation that is associated with the deaths of tens of thousands of patients and not be held accountable? The US health care culture still does not support the questioning of physician behavior.

Dr. Pronovost goes on describe the chasm that still exists between the culture of medical practice and the culture of science:

> … many physicians have not accepted that fallibilities are part of the human condition. Thus, when a nurse questions them, it causes embarrassment or shame. Clinicians are sometimes arrogant, believing they have all the answers, dismissing team input, responding aggressively when questioned. … autonomy becomes arrogance when actions are mindless and not mindful, when something is done simply because a physician demands it, when a clinician does not learn from mistakes, and when experimentation occurs without a clear rationale or testable hypothesis. Too often autonomy is mindless and driven by arrogance.[274]

Changing the hierarchy of practitioners would be a necessary part of introducing scientific order and rigor to medical practice. This would involve focused, skills-based training that would be far less time-consuming and expensive than physician training. That change would reduce economic and social barriers to entry into medical practice. Underserved rural and inner-city communities would then increasingly find practitioners within their own inhabitants. Meeting the high standards of performance demanded by uniform credentialing standards, these practitioners would provide high quality care to underserved areas (if given sufficient resources and infrastructure). Moreover, those who entered the health professions would be free to expand the depth and

---

274 Pronovost P. Learning Accountability for Patient Outcomes. JAMA 304:2; 204-205 (July 14, 2010).

scope of their expertise as their talents and drive permit. Upward mobility would then become part of the caregiving professions, unlike the status quo, where few upward career paths exist for nurses and other non-physician practitioners (short of suspending their careers to undergo many years of physician training). In this regard, health care needs to become more like the commercial world. In that world a young person with limited education may ascend the corporate ladder, or build a small business into a large enterprise, without first acquiring expensive professional credentials. More innovation in health care delivery would occur if the health care workforce had more opportunity to pursue innovation and its rewards.

In addition to lack of upward mobility, the demoralizing, out-of-control conditions of medical practice harm the health care professions. These conditions deprive caregiving of many of the emotional, intellectual and financial rewards that it should naturally produce. The result is serious manpower shortages, especially in primary care. In other words, a large sector of the economy is deprived of the rewarding employment opportunities that it should generate in every community. By contrast, removing credential barriers and creating a secure system of defined inputs and continuous improvement would make the health professions far more attractive. The field would draw countless individuals with the characteristics needed to become compassionate and skillful practitioners. Indeed, the interpersonal qualities needed for primary care and the technical aptitudes needed for skill in medical procedures are more widely distributed than the narrow intellectual abilities demanded by physician training.[275] Thus the caregiving professions would have a large pool of talent to draw upon. The economy as a whole could benefit enormously at many levels.

One of the intellectual rewards of the caregiving professions is the opportunity to participate in continuous improvement of medical knowledge, technique and quality of care. (Indeed, this opportunity exists not only for practitioners but for many administrative workers, as Dr. Bartholomew's description of his work with his medical records technician suggests (see note 272).) In a reformed system, practitioners would be constantly exposed to the gaps between medical knowledge and the realities of individual patients. Moreover, all practitioners would have genuine expertise in whatever functions they are licensed to perform, and would constantly be required to maintain and improve that expertise. Medical practice and medical education would thus be inseparable.

---

275 See C.C. Weed, *The Philosophy, Use and Interpretation of Knowledge Couplers* (note 2 above), p. 14 ("We can also hope that medical education will at least select for and not against those people who care most deeply about alleviating the suffering of others").

This combination of learning and doing has pivotal importance. Consider the following description of what used to be one of the most successful manufacturing companies in the world:

> The essence of Toyota's manufacturing philosophy [is] that it doesn't distinguish between learning and doing. ... Toyota wants its employees always to wonder how they may do things better. If a worker isn't learning, he isn't doing his job. As Steven Spear and H. Kent Bowen of Harvard Business School wrote in the Harvard Business Review, "The key is to understand that the Toyota Production System creates a community of scientists...the Toyota system actually stimulates workers and managers to engage in the kind of experimentation that is widely recognized as the cornerstone of a learning organization.[276]

The linkage between learning and doing is important not just for activities like manufacturing and health care but for reform of education itself. And it is important for educating not just health care workers but patients, the consumers of care who need to learn to manage their own health.

---

276 Jonah Lehrer, How We Know: What do an algebra teacher, Toyota and a classical musician have in common? *Seed* (Sep. 2006), http://www.seedmagazine.com/news/2006/07/how_we_know.php?page=all&p=y.

IX.
Education and the Role of the Patient/Consumer

A. Autonomy

If patient-consumers are to manage their own health, they need to learn to interact with the health care system autonomously, very much as they learn to navigate the transportation system. They need to face the central role of their own behaviors in determining their health. They need to access and understand their own medical records, and to use software tools for coupling medical knowledge with their own data. They need to understand their biological uniqueness and why it means they must manage their own care. They need to see the chasm between the non-system of care in which physicians are educated and the trustworthy, transparent system of care that could be built for their own use. They need to learn why they cannot rely on physicians to recall or apply established medical knowledge, nor rely on that knowledge to comprehend their own uniqueness, nor rely on the marketing of vendors as a source of knowledge, nor rely on physicians to make inherently personal decisions that belong to them alone. To enable this kind of autonomy, they need a trustworthy guidance system, a system of order and transparency that constantly incorporates new knowledge and harvests user experiences.

All of this has been largely absent from the status quo. The historical roots of the status quo are traced by Paul Starr. Comparing attitudes towards medical science during the Jacksonian and Progressive periods, Starr writes:

> In each period, the continuing, unresolved tensions between the nation's democratic culture and its capitalist economy became particularly acute. Both the Jacksonians and Progressives esteemed science, but they understood it in different ways. The Jacksonians saw science as knowledge that could be widely and easily diffused, while the Progressives were reconciled to its complexity and inaccessibility.[277]

---

277 Starr P., *The Social Transformation of American Medicine* (New York: Basic Books, 1982), p. 140.

The outcome in the 20th Century was that "American faith in democratic simplicity and common sense yielded to a celebration of science and efficiency."[278] This involved acceptance of professional authority, a "retreat from private judgment" and a "general decline of confidence in the ability of laymen to deal with their own physical and personal problems."[279] Patients thus became increasingly dependent on licensed, expert professionals for information, judgment and skillful performance.

The Flexner report reinforced this trend by linking the medical profession more closely to the university. That linkage was crucial, because the university has never faced up to the problem of distributing intellectual wealth. Viewing personal intellect as the primary vehicle for retrieving and applying knowledge, universities focus on the development of intellect. Never fully embracing the legacy of Francis Bacon, universities have neglected alternatives to intellect as a vehicle for transmitting and applying knowledge to human needs.

The outcome for medicine is that university-trained experts have always been seen as repositories of medical knowledge and the capacity for applying it. Perpetuating this cultural authority is the legal authority conferred on physicians by state medical practice acts (see part VIII.B).

This culture of dependence on medical experts is now beginning to break down. The Internet is lessening patient dependence on physicians for information and judgment. Simple, inexpensive devices for diagnostic testing and monitoring further lessen the physician role in some medical procedures. But these technological advances are not enough to create the system of care needed by patients and practitioners alike. The new diagnostic devices, for example, generate detailed data that must be organized in the medical record. The data must be coupled with medical knowledge from the Internet and elsewhere, and medical knowledge must be distilled and organized for that purpose.

Adopting these and other necessary elements of a system of care makes possible a fundamental shift of decision making responsibility from practitioners to patients.[280] In this scenario, patients are autonomous users of the system of care. Rather than being dependent on expert providers for information and judgment, patients choose the services they need, consulting with trusted practitioners as they wish and employing experts as needed for delivery of those

---

278 *Ibid.*

279 *Ibid.*, p. 141.

280 The following discussion draws on Weed, LL, "Introduction: Scientific principles that tell us why people must manage their own health care," in *Your Health Care and How To Manage It* (Essex Junction, VT: Essex Publishing Co., Inc., 1975), reproduced in Appendix B; Weed LL., et al., *Knowledge Coupling*, note 2 above, pp. 12-14, 105, 109-11, 193-205; Part II and IV.C of Opening the black box of clinical judgment, note 2 above.

services. Recall our analogy with the transportation system (see part I). Recall further the distinction between the two stages of decision making (see part III.A): first, identifying individualized options and evidence; second, choosing among the options. In both stages, the physician's role would be subordinate—in the first stage subordinate to information tools, and in the second stage subordinate to the patient's judgment, values and self-knowledge.

Without a total system of care, this shift in decision making authority from physicians to patients will not occur. What may occur instead is a reform scenario commonly discussed—that providers would become better organized to deliver "patient-centered care" through some form of "medical home." Patients would use information tools but still depend on physicians to guide decisions and coordinate care. Physicians would delegate "preference-sensitive" decisions to patients, but the physicians would identify those decisions and define the options presented. This dependence on physicians would seem unavoidable, because patients would lack a system of care in which they could function autonomously. The tacit knowledge of disease that physicians acquire from their experience would seem like indispensable expertise to physicians and patients alike, because neither physicians or patients would have a system exposing the limitations of that knowledge and experience. In short, this scenario views patient-consumers as largely passive beneficiaries of care chosen under the guidance of the physician experts who deliver it.

As between the two scenarios just described, only the first one (patient autonomy) is viable in the two basic situations that matter most: where the patient must face genuine medical uncertainty, and where the patient must cope with chronic disease. In situations of uncertainty, the patient faces a set of choices, with substantial evidence for and against each choice based on the details specific to his or her own case. The physician cannot be relied upon to identify the individually relevant options and evidence without the right informational infrastructure. Once that infrastructure is available, reliance on the physician radically diminishes. The patient's private judgment should control, as trade-offs are recognized, ambiguities assessed and choices made. The choices are inherently personal.

The other situation in which to compare the two scenarios (patient autonomy vs. patient dependence) involves cases of chronic disease, where the economic burdens of health care on society are concentrated. These cases start with great uncertainty, but often what needs to be done becomes reasonably clear from careful investigation and planning. Then the issue is execution, feedback and adjustment. Throughout these processes, the patient's role is decisive. Imagine the patient as the driver of a car (to borrow an analogy from Norbert Wiener, who used it to illustrate the importance of feedback in complex behaviors). No one can drive a car blindfolded by listening to directions from a passenger. This is so even if the passenger is more knowledgeable about driving the vehicle or navigating the route. That expertise in the passenger is no substitute for the driver's personally receiving and responding to visual feedback while driving. So it is in the care of chronic disease. There can be no substitute for the patient's taking on the responsibility to exercise private judgment. That is, the patient must personally learn about his or her condition, consider the pros and cons of therapeutic alternatives (including behavior changes), choose among those alternatives in light of personal values and circumstances, act on the choice, get feedback on the results and make corrective adjustments over time. The physician cannot be sure of making the same decision that the patient would make. Even if the physician's decision is the same, it cannot have the same psychological effect as the patient's making the decision for himself. It is the patient, not the physician, who must live with the risks, the pain, the trade-offs, the effort and time that the decision may entail. In Hayek's terms (see note 133 above), the patient is the one "closest to the subject matter of the decision," with "intimate knowledge" of the disease as uniquely experienced by that individual (see Appendix B for further discussion). It is true that some patients are without the mental capacity for decision making. In those situations, family members and not the physician are positioned to act on the patient's behalf.

The course of a chronic disease depends on numerous variables, none of which the practitioner personally experiences, most of which the practitioner does not control and some of which the practitioner is not aware. In diabetes, for example, blood glucose levels depend on not only insulin levels but also diet, exercise, emotion, medications, infections and co-existing medical problems, among other variables. The patient has more knowledge and control of some of these variables than the provider ever will. Managing chronic conditions demands keeping track of these variables over time and examining them for medically significant patterns and relationships. The provider's expertise is limited to textbook generalizations and limited personal experience with *other* patients, neither of which is sufficient to cope with detailed data and arrive at individualized decisions for the patient at hand. Those decisions require expertise that resides only in that patient, feedback that only the patient can recognize and act on, and external tools that the patient has more time and personal incentive to carefully use than most providers.[281] The patient feels the effects

---

281 "In some delivery systems, patients can view their own test results (including abnormal ones) online without having to wait for the physician to 'release' them. Many clinicians have already had a patient notice an important abnormality that they had overlooked in a laboratory

of the disease and its treatments, and quickly sees correlations between those subjective symptoms and detailed data on physiological parameters. Without any formal education, the patient is in the best position to observe these correlations. To that extent, information asymmetry exists in favor of the patient, not the expert provider. What the patient needs is not the broad, sophisticated scientific understanding of a physician but rather a basic understanding of principles and data that bear specifically on choosing among individually relevant options. And it is not unusual to see patients who develop more than this basic understanding. For example, diabetics of long-standing whose disease is well-controlled are frequently more knowledgeable about the disease and their personal version of it than their physicians.

Most of all, the patient is the one who must summon the resolve to make the behavior changes that so often are involved in coping with chronic disease. If the patient does not feel responsible for deciding what has to be done and is not heavily involved in developing the informational basis of that decision, then very often the result is "noncompliance" with doctors' decisions. Noncompliance may or may not be appropriate, depending on the situation. The point is that if patients are equipped to become decision makers, the problem of noncompliance with their doctors' decisions is transformed into a problem of personal commitment to their own decisions. Patients will be more committed to their own, informed decisions than to decisions made for them by experts.[282]

Patient autonomy in this scenario does not mean that patients make difficult medical decisions on their own, without involvement of others. Rather, as in other areas of their lives, patients exercise personal judgment after turning to (or being confronted by) trusted parties (family, friends, co-workers, practitioners) who provide dialogue, guidance, feedback and emotional support. Some patients will still choose to defer heavily to practitioner judgments, especially where the issues are more technical than personal, but that deference should be the patient's choice.

Patient autonomy does not mean that patients may choose whatever medical care they wish without regard to cost or medical necessity. Patients, providers, and third party payers should not be able to impose medical or financial decisions on each other unilaterally. Checks and balances are needed, including a system for adjudicating disputes. But the standards for adjudication must recognize the

---

result; that experience will probably become more common as patients gain broader access to their medical records." Gandhi T, Lee T. Patient Safety beyond the Hospital, note 6 above.

282 Factors like these explain the research findings that patient involvement in decision making improves health outcomes. See Berwick D., What Patient-Centered Should Mean: Confessions of an Extremist, *Health Affairs*, May 19, 2009 (see the discussion at notes 12-14) available at http://content.healthaffairs.org/cgi/content/full/hlthaff.28.4.w555/DC1.

patient's central role. Deference to patient judgment, as distinguished from the judgments of providers or third parties, will lead to more rational decisions. For patients, unlike providers, medical care is an unfortunate necessity, not a source of income and not a career interest to pursue. The patient's incentive is to obtain the best care *but no more*. And the best care is often not the most expensive care.

This is not to deny that some "professional patients" seek more care than they medically need, due to psychological issues. But such patients are the exception, not the rule. Coping with them requires a system of corrective checks and balances—the same protection we need against dysfunctional behaviors by providers and payers, and the same system we need to guide normal behaviors by all parties.[283] Insurance protection, for example, should enable patients to individually balance cost against benefit in a rational way, protecting them from serious financial harm while still giving them a financial stake, both short-term and long-term, in their own decisions and their own behaviors.[284]

For patients to acquire the necessary understanding and become equipped to cope with their chronic conditions, decision making processes must move from Karl Popper's World 2 to World 3, from personal recall, knowledge and judgment to highly organized records, including graphs and flowsheets for organizing objective data, plus decision support tools that bring objective knowledge to bear on this data in a usable manner, all used jointly by patients practitioners. Consulting with practitioners, patients themselves can use decision support tools to identify options and evidence. They can use medical records to discern their own unique patterns of response, to see what works and what doesn't work. And others can use these records to confront irresponsible patients with feedback on the medical consequences of their own actions or inaction.[285] External tools in World 3 thus provide concrete instruments for capitalizing upon the personal knowledge and motivation of patients, very much as the price system in a market economy capitalizes upon the personal knowledge and motivation of market participants.

As between the two scenarios outlined above, the second scenario (practitioners in control of "patient-centered" care) is more compatible with

---

283 Recall from part I our discussion of corrective feedback loops. These maintain compatibility between common purposes and the actions taken, individually and collectively, in pursuit of those purposes.

284 This kind of balancing is the purpose of consumer-driven arrangements. Recall from part II.B.2.d our distinction between consumer-driven *spending* arrangements and consumer-driven *care*. The pros and cons of alternative consumer-driven spending arrangements are beyond the scope of this book.

285 For two examples of this kind of interaction using problem-oriented medical records, see Dr. Ken Bartholomew's descriptions in *Knowledge Coupling* (cited in note 129 above), p. 265.

the current medical culture, rooted in World 2. But the first scenario (patient autonomy) is more compatible with the movement to World 3 made possible by modern information technology. Patients would naturally use the system of care in World 3 as the primary source of information for decision making. The question remains, however—where do patients turn for outside guidance and judgment? Most people do not make important personal decisions based on purely private judgment. Most people rely in part on dialogue with others. Many physicians provide that dialogue, making enormous contributions to their patients' lives in the process. But there is no reason for physicians to monopolize the role of a trusted party for dialogue. Although physicians may have relevant experience with other patients who have had the "same" disease," that experience may also mislead, because each patient is unique. Moreover, not all physicians have (and many non-physician practitioners *do* have) the interpersonal skills or temperament to participate in dialogue effectively. Nor do physicians acquire any special expertise in that role from their medical training. Nor do they often have sufficient time for a real dialogue. Nor do they often have a sufficiently close personal relationship with patients. Various other professionals who specialize in counseling roles are often better suited than physicians, and better positioned in patient lives, to engage in dialogue about medical problems.

More fundamentally, as our analogy with the transportation system suggests, dependence on professionals is very often not what patients want or need. In many situations, the best source of guidance, feedback and emotional support may not be professionals but rather family, friends and colleagues who are already part of the patient's life. And *other* patients may be the best source of the expertise and support most relevant to a patient's medical needs. Online communities oriented to particular diseases are full of people who have developed deep knowledge about their condition and who have devoted themselves to dialogue with others. Moreover, those communities are often the best way to locate others whose condition is the most similar to the patient's own.[286]

In short, patients themselves are the greatest untapped resource in the health care system. There is one for every member of the population. And they are the best positioned, in terms of personal knowledge and motivation, to manage chronic disease and make decisions in the face of genuine medical uncertainty. But for the health care system to take full advantage of this resource, the educational system will need to change.

---

286 See, for example, www.patientslikeme.com

B. Education

If health care is to be patient-centered and consumer-driven, if patient-consumers are to become autonomous, if they are to apply medical knowledge to their own medical problems, then they as well as their practitioners need medical education. That education should begin in early childhood, a time when regular contact with health problems and the health care system naturally occur. But the education that is required is profoundly different from traditional schooling. This is not because health care is somehow less suited to traditional schooling than other fields. It is because traditional schooling is so often unsuited to genuine education in any field. [287]

Recall our discussion (part VIII.A) of how medical education fails to integrate basic science with clinical practice, and the toxic effects on students. T. S. Eliot similarly criticized formal education in general for failure to integrate abstract ideas with students' personal realities:

> the ordinary processes of society which constitute education for the ordinary man ... consist largely in the acquisition of impersonal ideas which obscure what we really are and feel, what we really want, and what really excites our interest. It is of course not the actual information acquired, but the conformity which the accumulation of knowledge is apt to impose, that is harmful. [288]

In the same vein, Alfred North Whitehead identified "the problem of keeping knowledge alive, of preventing it from becoming inert" as "the central problem of all education." [289] Recognizing this problem, John Dewey analyzed it in terms of the need to connect language and ideas with experience:

---

287 Much of the discussion here is adapted from *Knowledge Coupling*, note 2 above, pp. 9-12, 14-19, 198, 205, 209-16.

288 T.S. Eliot, "Blake," in *The Sacred Wood: Essays on Poetry and Criticism.* 1922, available at http://www.bartleby.com/200/sw13.html. A related point was made by the cognitive psychologist Robyn Dawes in the context of discussing the pitfalls of automatic, associative thinking (as distinguished from controlled thinking—deliberate hypothesizing of possibilities). Dawes argued that "education does not necessarily help" avoid those pitfalls of associative thinking. "The reason is that so much of what passes for education consists of memorizing connections between words, phrases and images. These words phrases and images may or may not have any connection to external reality." Dawes, note 127 above, p. 79. Similarly, Eliot sees that formal education involves acquiring impersonal ideas that may or may not have any connection to *internal* reality. Eliot goes on to discuss the limitations of Blake's informal self-education, which was well connected to his internal reality but insufficiently connected to an external "framework of accepted and traditional ideas."

289 Whitehead, A. *The Aims of Education and Other Essays* (Macmillan, 1929). Whitehead defined "inert ideas" as "ideas that are merely received into the mind, without being utilized, or tested, or thrown into fresh combinations" (p. 1).

words, symbols come to take the place of ideas. The substitution is more subtle because *some* meaning is recognized. But we are very easily trained to be content with a minimum of meaning and to fail to note how restricted our perception of the relations which confer significance. We get so thoroughly used to a kind of pseudo-idea, a half perception, that we are not aware how half-dead our mental action is, and how much keener and more extensive our observations and idea would be if we formed them under conditions of a vital experience which required us to use judgment: to hunt for the connections of the thing dealt with.[290]

Solving the problem of inert knowledge drove Dewey's approach to education. Recall his view that knowledge should be a by-product of activity (see note 244). Dewey's "mission was to 'reinstate experience into education' ... to make education seem indivisible from action. Dewey's insights are needed now more than ever. ... Unfortunately, in the age of standardized testing, US schools have given up on Dewey's experiential approach ..."[291]

Abstracting knowledge from the problem-solving activities to which it should relate has damaging effects at many levels. One effect is that formal education becomes focused unduly on personal intellect. Cultivating a narrow range of intellectual skills and temperaments that foster academic success, the culture of education takes interpersonal skills for granted, and devalues manual skills.[292] And it fails to instill the intellectual behaviors and perspectives that foster effective problem-solving (see part V).

In particular, traditional schooling fails to instill high standards of achievement. In most schooling, time is the constant and achievement the variable—precisely the opposite of what true education demands. Students are allotted a fixed amount of time to learn and then permitted to pass exams and courses with a B or C or worse. Inevitably, given the widely varying abilities and inclinations of individual students, not many will have the experience of passing courses at a high level of achievement. This tolerance of lesser achievement is especially harmful when learning is cumulative, that is, when success at one level requires understanding of the material from an earlier level.

---

290 Dewey, *Democracy and Education*, note 244 above, p. 144. Dewey elsewhere emphasizes that "'vital experience" includes social connections. He stated "the principle that things gain meaning by being used in a shared experience of joint action." *Ibid.*, p. 16. With respect to language, "its use should be more vital and fruitful by having its normal connection with shared activities." *Ibid.*, p. 38.

291 Jonah Lehrer, How We Know, note 276 above.

292 See Crawford M. The Case for Working With Your Hands, *New York Times Magazine*, May 24, 2009, available at http://www.nytimes.com/2009/05/24/magazine/24labor-t.html?_r=1 (adapted from *Shop Class as Soulcraft: An Inquiry Into the Value of Work* (Penguin Press, 2009)).

Failure to enforce high standards of quality arises from the premise that schooling should instill a fixed core of knowledge, as distinguished from a core of behavior. Teaching high standards of intellectual behavior and teaching a fixed core of knowledge are mutually exclusive when a fixed time is allotted to achieving these goals. One of the three variables (time spent, amount covered and degree of mastery) has to be held constant at a high level, and that constant should be the degree of mastery. Students would differ in the *amount* they master and the *speed* with which they do so, but not in the degree of mastery they attain.

Mastery of a core of knowledge should not be the goal of education—especially in an era when knowledge is constantly becoming obsolete and when information technology confers rapid access to more knowledge than anyone can learn and more processing power than anyone's mind possesses. The goal should be mastering the behaviors involved in applying knowledge to solve problems effectively and efficiently.

Because these principles are ignored, many students pass through 12 or more years of schooling without ever experiencing mastery, while constantly undergoing invidious comparisons to the best students. This system is harmful even for those best students, for they may acquire elitist attitudes, superficial understanding[293] and misplaced confidence that their academic proficiency will translate into effective problem solving. For less successful students, schooling is too often experienced as a caste system rather than a vehicle for personal development. Many students emerge from their schooling with their natural abilities undeveloped and their natural optimism defeated. To fight back, some adopt an attitude of disdain towards education and intellect. These reactions to formal education are like the reaction of dying canaries in a coal mine—highly sensitive indicators of toxic conditions. In varying degrees, many students are left without the capacities and confidence that only achievement can confer and without the expanded horizons that only education can provide.

Above (part VIII.A.2) we argued that the only workable approach to medical education for practitioners is careful engagement of students in patient care itself, so that students *use* medical knowledge rather than learn it in the abstract. This concept can and should be generalized, as John Dewey envisioned, to all education. Now that information technology can be employed to capture knowledge in maximally usable form, the futility of learning knowledge in the abstract is more apparent and more avoidable than ever before. Using knowledge involves coupling a current problem situation with prior experiences of others who faced similar situations. This process of making connections is

---

293 See note 244 above.

accomplished far more easily, comprehensively, and reliably with some form of knowledge coupling software than with traditional texts and limited personal knowledge. Dewey conceived knowledge in these terms:

> knowledge is a perception of those connections of an object which determine its applicability in a given situation. ... We respond to [an event's] *connections* and not simply to the immediate occurrence. ... An ideally perfect knowledge would represent such a network of interconnections that any past experience would offer a point of advantage from which to get at the problem presented in a new experience.[294]

Conceiving knowledge in these terms leads naturally to using some form of knowledge coupling tools to build and navigate a network of interconnections. That network would capture much of what we now regard as personal experience and expertise, connecting those resources to problem situations as they are encountered by inexperienced non-experts for the first time. And that in turn could lead to a new form of education, where students would be judged on their personal effectiveness in using network connections to solve real problems, rather than their personal displays of disconnected knowledge.

Connecting education with real-world problem situations, where solutions have value to someone, would have beneficial effects at many levels. We have already discussed how actual problem-solving teaches students the fallibility of received "knowledge" (see part VIII.A above). Moreover, as compared to rote learning, and even as compared to problems contrived for educational purposes, real problems (practical or theoretical) mobilize in students their natural curiosity, their collaborative instincts, their willingness to question authority, and their desire to engage in productive, meaningful activity. Students would be spared the stultifying years in schools that have so little meaning for so many of them. For students from harmful home or community environments where problems seem insoluble, the educational process could become a haven, where problems *are* soluble and personal development takes root.

In a prophetic work, *Deschooling Society*, Ivan Illich argued that schooling is a ritual with only a tenuous relationship to genuine education. A "major illusion on which the school system rests is that most learning is the result of teaching. Teaching, it is true, may contribute to certain kinds of learning under certain

---

294 *Democracy and Education*, note 244 above, p. 340 (emphasis in original). Elsewhere Dewey explains:: "All authorities agree that that discernment of relationships is the genuinely intellectual matter; hence, the educative matter. The failure arises in supposing that relationships can become perceptible without experience ..." *Ibid.*, p. 144.

circumstances. But most people acquire most of their knowledge outside of school..."[295] Illich distinguished skill-learning from "education in the exploratory and creative use of skills." Learning of specific skills can benefit greatly from planned instruction by teachers, but only strongly motivated students will derive this benefit. Their motivation usually arises from some outside engagement in the problem for which the skills offer a solution. Similarly, education for inventive and creative behavior relies on relationships among "individuals starting from their own, unresolved questions." These relationships differ from those in academia. "In schools, including universities, most resources are spent to purchase the time and motivation of a limited number of people to take up predetermined problems in a ritually defined setting. The most radical alternative to school would be a network or service which gave each man the same opportunity to share his current concern with others motivated by the same concern."[296]

These concepts are central to the problem of educating patient-consumers, from childhood, to become autonomous users of the health care system and careful stewards of their own health. The key is to expose them from early childhood to a trustworthy, transparent, disciplined system of care. In that environment, children will naturally learn that they have personal knowledge of and control over their own health that no expert provider could ever have. They will naturally learn personal responsibility for improving their own health and for navigating the health care system autonomously. Again, John Dewey expressed the key principle: "the only way in which adults consciously control the kind of education which the immature get is by controlling the environment in which they act, and hence think and feel."[297]

Dewey advocated an approach to childhood education rooted in the child's personal experience and environment. Yet, Dewey's experiential approach never entered the educational mainstream.[298] One reason for this may be the

---

295 Illich, I. *Deschooling Society* (New York: Harper & Row, 1970), p. 12. See also John Taylor Gatto, "Against School, *Harper's Magazine*, Sep. 2003 (pp. 33-38); John Taylor Gatto, *Dumbing Us Down: The Hidden Curriculum of Compulsory Schooling* (New Society Publishers, 1992, original edition).

296 *Ibid.*, pp. 17-19.

297 Dewey, J., *Democracy and Education*, note 241 above, p. 18.

298 Labaree D. "Limits on the Impact of Educational Reform: The Case of Progressivism and U.S. Schools, 1900-1950," Nov. 30, 2007, at http://www.stanford.edu/~dlabaree/publications/Monte_Verita_Paper.pdf. Greater acceptance has occurred for the educational approach established by Dewey's contemporary, Maria Montessori. Montessori education shares important elements with Dewey's approach. One recent study has found Montessori education to have outcomes superior to traditional education based on measures of cognitive/academic and social behavioral skills. Lillard A. and Else-Quest N., Evaluating Montessori Education, *Science*, 313:1893-94 (29 Sep. 2006). See also Matthews, J., Montessori, Now 100, Goes Mainstream; Washington *Post*, January 2, 2007, available at http://www.washingtonpost.com/

apparent difficulty of developing broad and deep educational experiences out of the limited personal experiences and environments of children.

But it is not hard to imagine how an approach to education centered on medicine could offer enormous breadth and depth while remaining connected with students' personal experience. Every child has a natural interest in the workings of his or her own body and mind. Each child encounters health care—not only the care each receives but also the care provided to family and friends, and the practitioners who provide it. This exposure could lead to exploring the skills practitioners acquire, the knowledge they apply, the discipline they develop, the technologies they use, the institutions they work in, the economics involved. Education could involve participation in caregiving activities, working with patients and the people who care for them at institutions in the local community. Education could involve learning the principles, skills and behaviors required for maintaining personal health, making informed medical decisions, and coping with health problems, all in the context of witnessing the health problems and health behaviors of others. Education could involve exploring the science, the countless vocational skills, the psychological dimensions and the larger social and economic issues connected with health, disease and medical care.

Education centered on medicine would have the depth and breadth that Whitehead argued is essential: "Let the main ideas which are introduced into a child's education be few and important, and let them be thrown into every combination possible. The child should make them his own, and should understand their application here and now in the circumstances of his actual life." Education of this kind could connect learning by doing, learning from personal experiences and learning from the writings of others about their experiences—learning that would reach many students whom the current educational system cuts off from their own potential.[299]

The time may come when we look back on schooling in its present form as a misguided approach to education, almost as we look back on alchemy and astrology in the time of Francis Bacon as misguided approaches to science. Like the experimental method of science, education must be rooted in a disciplined

---

wp-dyn/content/article/2007/01/01/AR2007010100742.html; Haines A., Baker K., Kahn D., Optimal Developmental Outcomes: The Social, Moral, Cognitive, and Emotional Dimensions of a Montessori Education; NAMTA Journal 25:2, Spring, 2000; 26:1, Winter, 2001; 28:1, Winter 2003; available at www.montessori-namta.org/NAMTA/PDF%20files/Outcomes.pdf. This article discusses, among other things, Dewey's and Montessori's shared concern with real-life occupations for learners; "an occupation leads naturally to a search for contextual knowledge" (p. 31).

299 *The Aims of Education and Other Essays,* note 289, p. 2.

process of trial, error and feedback, making connections between theory and practice, the mind and external reality. In education, this process must be closely tied to the learner's personal realities, internal and external. Yet, the culture of medicine and the culture of education are still occupied with the disconnected mind and impersonal ideas, like the universities and the received bodies of thought that Bacon faced 400 years ago. Bacon envisioned better connections among the mind, the external world, and objective knowledge, using the experimental method of science. But to arrive at this new vision, Bacon had to overcome an entrenched and stifling world view. In Loren Eisely's words:

> The real problem was to break with the dead hand of the traditional past, to free latent intellectual talent, to arrest and touch with hope the popular mind, to carry word of that which lay beyond the scope of the isolated individual thinker; namely, to dramatize ... the invention of the experimental method—the invention of inventions, the door to man's control of his own future."[300]

As John Dewey recognized, "the progress of experimental science ... has demonstrated that there is no such thing as genuine knowledge and fruitful understanding except as the offspring of doing."[301] Whether this principle is embraced will determine the direction in which health care and education evolve.

The direction we take remains to be seen. We are the agents of our own evolution. We must break with the dead hand of the past, if we are to open new doors to control of our own futures.

---

300 Eisely, L., *Francis Bacon and the Modern Dilemma* (Lincoln: University of Nebraska Press 1962), p. 22.

301 See note 244 above.

APPENDIX A

Analysis of two clinical trials

Lister's was an innovation not altogether easy to imitate. It was a complicated technique, not a standardized formula, and it was therefore essential to read Lister's descriptions of the method very carefully and in their entirety. There is ample evidence that this was often not done. ... But the difficulty found by many in doing what Lister recommended, and the consequent 'failures' that were held to prove the uselessness of antisepsis, were bound up with a second difficulty. This was, that antiseptic surgery depended on a theory. Those who did not understand or accept the theory, and who nevertheless tried to follow antiseptic procedures were liable to constant mistakes, because they were not guided by the rationale of what they were doing.

— *A. J. Youngson*[302]

This Appendix reviews two studies of PKC Corporation knowledge coupling software. Both of these studies compare a group of providers and patients using the software with a control group not using the software. For reasons discussed in Part IV.D above, studies of this kind have limited value. Nevertheless, we review them here because these studies may be of interest to many readers, and because of their conceptual significance.

1. The VA Study

Goolsby J. Implementation and Evaluation of PKC© Software at the James A. Haley Veterans' Hospital in Tampa, Florida, February 16, 2001, available at http://www.pkc. com/papers/VA_tampa_report.pdf.[303]

This study involved a pilot project implementing PKC knowledge coupling software for managing diabetes. The study was intended to (1) "determine what

---

302 Youngson, A. *The Scientific Revolution in Victorian Medicine* (Holmes & Meier ,1979), p. 216 (from Chapter 12, entitled "The Fight for New Ideas," which provides a valuable analysis of resistance to innovation).

303 This study is discussed in "Beyond guidelines: Tool arms physicians with critical knowledge at the point of care," *Disease Management Advisor*, January 2002, pp. 9—12.

was necessary to implement the software," and (2) "examine the clinical efficacy and effectiveness of its use" (p. 2). Two patient cohorts were compared, one serving as the intervention group and one serving as the control group.

The study analyzed use of the software module (Coupler) for diabetes management (Diabetes Coupler). This Coupler is designed to be used in conjunction with a Coupler for taking patient histories (History Coupler). Accordingly, the study design required providers using the Diabetes Coupler for the intervention group also to use the History Coupler. Providers in the control group used neither the Diabetes or History Couplers. Beyond this, the basic elements of the study were as follows:

Selection of intervention and control groups. Providers in the intervention group were new, first-year resident physicians, who began work on July 1, 2000 at the hospital's Internal Medicine Clinic, where the study was conducted. New residents were selected for the intervention group because they "were less entrenched and could be controlled more than attending physicians. ... it was made non-negotiable to the resident physicians that (1) the output of the coupler would be used and (2) the level of medical care prescribed would be followed" (p. 11).

Patients were assigned to the intervention and control groups (38 in each group) as follows:

- The patients assigned to the intervention group were those attending the Internal Medicine Clinic on three specified weekday afternoons. The resident physicians in the Clinic at those half-days were isolated during their Clinic attendance from other resident physicians and patients not in the intervention group.

- Patients were assigned to the control group by randomly selecting every 38th patient from all diabetic patients attending the Internal Medicine Clinic during the seven half-days of the week other than the half-days on which the intervention group was in the Clinic.

In order to examine whether the patients in these groups were comparable, the two groups were compared statistically with respect to age, weight, height, body mass index and the five variables (see below) used to measure the patient outcomes, based on data immediately preceding the intervention. The two groups were found to be statistically equivalent by these measures (p. 16). In addition, the groups were similar in frequency of cardiovascular and renal diagnoses (74% of the intervention group and 71% of the control group had one or more of five enumerated conditions, pp. 18-19). For the two groups combined, "the majority of the diabetic patients studied here were elderly [the mean age was 65½] and critically ill, due to their severe cardiac, vascular and renal disease" (p. 27).

Intervention procedures. For the intervention group, patients completed the History Coupler, a member of the intervention team completed the Diabetes Coupler, the patient's medication and medical records were reviewed, and current vital signs were taken. After completion of this process, the assigned resident physician saw the patient. The study described this initial encounter as follows (pp. 20-21):

When the patient first entered the treatment room, the assigned resident physician had available on the computer screen in that room the relevant findings of the patient's history in a concise, organized format (as opposed to the normal thick file folder of indecipherable notes), the results of the disease Coupler and the patient's current status based on [the VA's computerized medical record system]. The resident physician would then review the output with the patient, along with any other interested parties in the room, such as family members, if the patient so desired. Based on the output, the physician would prescribe treatment and provide print-outs of information and knowledge contained in the software.

Variables selected to measure intervention effect. The study compared the intervention and control groups with respect to five clinical goals established by the American Diabetes Association:

1. Systolic blood pressure < 130 mm Hg

2. Diastolic blood pressure < 80 mm Hg

3. Hemoglobin A_{1c} < 7%

4. Microalbuminuria < 30 mg albumin /g creatinine

5. Serum LDL Cholesterol < mg/dL

"Each of these standards, or performance measures, when unmet, indicates a condition that needs attention. Therapeutic interventions that are relatively straightforward can be easily provided for each" (p. 14).

Measured variables before and after intervention. The results of the study (pp. 21-26) were decisive. With respect to four of the five measures examined, the new residents in the intervention group attained results clearly superior to those of the experienced physicians in the control group. Specifically, over the seven month time period:

- Systolic blood pressure for the intervention group decreased by 10.3%, from well above to well below the recommended maximum level. For the control group, systolic blood pressure *increased*, starting well above the recommended level and leaving the patients 4.2% worse than that at the end.

- Diastolic blood pressure for the intervention group decreased by 10.8% (from 8% below the recommended level to 18.5% below). For the control group, diastolic blood pressure failed to decrease significantly.

- In testing for microalbuminuria, the proportion of patients for whom testing was done correctly (see pp. 22-24) increased from 24% to 100% in the intervention group, compared to an increase from 8% to 32% in the control group. Moreover, with respect to actually detecting patients with microalbuminuria, 12 such patients (32%) were detected in the intervention group, compared with only one (3%) in the control group. (See pages 22-24 of the study for details.) These patients were given appropriate therapy.

- For Hemoglobin A_{1c}, results were marginally better for the intervention group than for the control group, but the difference was not statistically significant. Neither group attained the standard of care.

- LDL cholesterol levels for the intervention group decreased by 9.1%, starting with patients 13.38% above the recommended maximum level (100 mg/dL) and ending with those patients 3.47% above that level. For the control group, LDL cholesterol levels *increased* by 3.4%, starting with patients 2.86% above the recommended level and ending with those patients 6.37% above that level. The difference between the two groups was statistically significant.

The following table (p. 26) summarizes the results in relation to the standard of care for the five measures:

Condition	Standard of Care	Intervention Pre	Intervention Post	Control Pre	Control Post	Significance P<
Systolic BP mmHg	< 130	139.3	124.9	136.0	141.7	.0001
Diastolic BP mmHg	< 80	73.8	65.8	70.74	70.16	.022
Microalbu-minuria Test	Conducted correctly	24%	100%	8%	32%	.001
Microalbumin-uria Present	Diagnosis confirmed	3%	32%	0%	3%	.001
Hemoglobin A_{1c}, %	< 7	8.1	7.4	7.7	7.5	.08
LDL Choles-terol, mg/DL	< 100	113.4	103.5	102.9	106.4	.08

In short, substantial improvements in the measured variables occurred for the intervention group but not for the control group. Indeed, two of the measures in the control group worsened. Moreover, by the end of the study period, three of the five measured variables met or exceeded the standard of care in the intervention group. The control group did not attain the standard of care (except for one variable, diastolic blood pressure, where the control group started out above the standard of care but failed to improve). These disparities between the two groups suggest that the intervention caused the improvement.

Impact on outcomes. As the study points out (p. 27), the five variables, and the seven month time period, are insufficient to measure ultimate outcomes, medical or economic. But the American Diabetes Association has determined that the five measured variables are highly relevant to the quality of diabetes care and its ultimate outcomes, for reasons the study explains (pp. 26-27):

Reductions in systolic and diastolic blood pressures have been shown to ameliorate the deleterious effects of diabetes. ... The confirmed presence of microalbuminuria in diabetics indicates the impending progression of to overt diabetic nephropathy and, eventually, end-stage renal disease and a higher than otherwise risk of cardiovascular disease and premature death. In this study the physicians seldom ordered tests for microalbuminuria and, when they did so, they did not follow protocols dictated by the literature. The intervention led to 100% compliance and to the first diagnosis of microalbuminuria in eleven patients, who might otherwise have been missed. ...

... The medical literature would predict that the long-term prognosis for quality of life has been improved, for example, by the intervention's potential forestalling of amputations, heart disease, and the need for dialysis.

The study goes on to explain that the characteristics of this particular patient population heighten the significance of the results:

... the majority of patients studied here were elderly and critically ill due to their severe cardiac, vascular and renal disease. One can only speculate on how much better their current condition might be had they been receiving the best practice medical care, as delivered in the present intervention, throughout the past five or more years, a period when the medical literature was already recommending the same preventive steps that, owing to the development of the PKC software, the intervention group received in the present study. [pp. 27-28]

Although one can only speculate on *how much* better off the patients might have been, it is more than speculation to conclude that over time the intervention would have left them clearly better off:

... the ravages of diabetic complications are incremental. Middle-aged veterans with diabetes, therefore, especially those without complications yet, might well benefit from the medical advantages afforded by the PKC software even more than the elderly, especially those with complications already. [p. 28]

The high costs of diabetic complications suggest the economic impact would be commensurate with the medical impact. This is especially apparent with respect to the impact on testing for microalbuminuria. "If the eleven patients whose presence of microalbuminuria was undetected previously but was diagnosed in this study were to remain off dialysis for two years, the savings would be $880,000 [assuming dialysis costs of $40,000/year]. Extend those patients to all patients in the study, and the savings escalate to $1.6 million" (p. 28).

What conclusions can be drawn? None of the elements of this study suggest that its results are unrepresentative of what could be accomplished with other diabetic populations. Nevertheless, the study's brief duration (seven months), small size (76 patients), and limited scope (one clinic at one medical center) make extrapolations from its particular results quite uncertain.

Independently of its particular results, this study is significant because both its design and its limitations illuminate the concept of a total system of care. Two basic points need to be understood.

First, the five measured variables are not complete measures of quality, regardless of whether quality is conceived process or outcome terms. A physician could attend carefully to each of the five variables but overlook other many other important elements of care. Indeed, that kind of oversight is the predictable result of measuring only a few elements. What is needed is a total system for organizing all elements of care. That is precisely what knowledge coupling software and the problem-oriented medical record accomplish. The Diabetes Coupler, for example, is designed to collect hundreds of data points (including the five measures studied here) and then to match them with specifically relevant medical knowledge, in conjunction with using other Couplers and problem-oriented medical records, as part of a total system of care for all of the patient's medical problems. A total system of care addresses all of a patient's problems and all relevant elements of each problem. From this perspective, it is quite artificial to focus on a few variables or one medical problem. The artificiality is especially apparent in patients with chronic disease, who typically have multiple, interrelated problems.

The second (and related) point that needs to be understood about this study is that it does not isolate the effect of using the knowledge coupling software, because it does not exclude another relevant variable—the possibility that the intervention group physicians were driven to act on the patient needs revealed by the software, including the five selected quality measures. Indeed, this clearly occurred with respect to the microalbuminuria testing variable: "it was made no longer negotiable to measure microalbuminuria, which is why conformance levels reached 100%" (p. 33). No such demand was made on the control group physicians. More generally, the study specifically observes that the participating practitioners were not blinded to the intervention and, moreover, were "biased positively toward the success of the project. This latter limitation is particularly applicable to the project leaders, who volunteered to participate. Inferences about implementing the software in similar settings without leadership support cannot be made validly" (pp. 12-13).

A skeptic might thus argue that it was not the software tools but the motivations of the intervention group participants that led to the favorable results. On this view, the control group physicians might have achieved similar results without the software if they specifically directed their efforts at the five performance measures examined. In other words, on this view the control group and intervention group physicians should have been equalized so that the only difference between them was whether or not they employed the software.

This point of view ignores the fact that introducing the software is only one element of reforming the total system of care. The software is designed to be an integral part of a reformed system of care, not to be an add-on to the failed status quo. A reformed system includes scrutinizing whether practitioners act on patient needs revealed by software tools. Introducing the software tools without that scrutiny is pointless (just as building a solid foundation without sound construction of the rest of the building is pointless). In any event, there is no possibility of testing the effect of the software in isolation, because introducing the software inevitably changes other elements of the working environment in ways that affect ultimate outcomes.

Now, let us consider the study's conclusion. The authors concluded that "the intervention caused the differences in measures" during the study period "because measures in the control group did not move at all" during that period (p. 26). This conclusion holds if "the intervention" is defined to include not only using the software but other changes associated with its use. Those changes included "devis[ing] a system whereby care could be elevated to levels dictated by the state-of-the-art medical knowledge prescribed by the software" (p. 10). For example, the project leaders communicated their vision that acceptable standards of care were being redefined to exceed the previously accepted community level standard (p. 10). In addition, as noted above, the intervention group physicians were limited new residents who "were less entrenched and could be controlled more than attending physicians" (p. 11). More generally, the intervention sought to ensure "that the software could be tested in an environment conducive to its proper functioning" (p. 11).

In the "post hoc analysis" (p. 29), the authors considered how the software contributed to the results. Specifically, the study identified three ways in which using the software improved perceptions, motivations and actions of practitioners in the intervention group:

- The software led the project leaders and the participating practitioners to recognize the need for better care. Before the intervention, practitioners at the Internal Medicine Clinic believed that their diabetes care "meets or exceeds community and some national standards." This belief was supported by "high level accreditations and numerous documentation establishing high levels of care" (p. 8). When the leaders were exposed to knowledge coupling software, however, they hypothesized that the Clinic's diabetes care was less than optimal and that using the software could improve it.[304] "Without the software, the leaders would not have been cognizant of the standards [of care in the software] and would have been motivated only to provide the level of care that was traditionally provided, which has been shown here to be inadequate" (p. 33). The software similarly transformed the perceptions of its users in the intervention group. "The software conclusively convinced those involved that the care normally administered, although thought to be adequate if not superior, was actually less than possible and below the level deserved" by patients (p. 30).

- The software led practitioners to recognize that their personal knowledge about managing diabetes was inadequate. Resistance to the software was founded on beliefs that (1) personal knowledge of experienced physicians is sufficient (2) the detailed data collection entailed by the software's comprehensive knowledge base is not a worthwhile tradeoff. Experience with the software, however, changed both these beliefs.[305]

- In a section entitled "Creating a Community of Care Providers," the study describes how the software elicited expertise relevant to patient problems. "For example, … a staff Nephrologist and Chief of the Renal Disease and Hypertension Section in the Medical Service, was consulted on specific patients when complications arose and served as a consultant to the team on treating hypertension and microalbuminuria.[306] *These interactions*

---

304 Significantly, the project leaders' first exposure to knowledge coupling software involved a completely different kind of medical problem: diagnosis of a rare genetic condition. One of the project leaders, Dr. Willard Harris, was witnessing a demonstration of PKC's software. A colleague presented a case that multiple physicians had been unable to diagnose for two years, until a few days before, when a second-year resident determined that the patient suffered from acquired C-1-esterase inhibitor deficiency, a rare inherited disorder. The PKC executive giving the software demonstration was presented with the patient's symptoms but not the diagnosis. He entered the symptoms into a relevant Coupler. It immediately generated the correct diagnosis. See W. Ring, "Software Backstops Doctors to Cut Errors," *Los Angeles Times* (AP), June 11, 2000, http://articles.latimes.com/2000/jun/11/news/mn-39856.

305 "All the physicians and residents participating in the study learned tremendously from the experience and expanded their knowledge, even desiring to go beyond the software to learn and obtain additional information. Once they had become involved, the tradeoffs seemed more worthwhile to them, but overcoming the initial resistance is difficult" (p. 30). The statement about users' expanding their knowledge should not be misunderstood. The primary benefit gained in the tradeoff is *not* expanding personal knowledge nor learning additional information beyond the software. The primary benefit is to escape dependence on personal knowledge by continuously improving the knowledge embedded in the software. Feedback from users' personal knowledge, experience and research is one vital source of this continuous improvement in the software.

306 Here as with the preceding note, it is important to understand that relevant expertise

would never have occurred without the guidance and stimulus provided by the software." (Emphasis added). Crucially, the "care providers" with whom this dynamic occurred were not only physician experts but also patients themselves and their family members. To enlist their active involvement, they received printouts of the History and Diabetes Coupler output:

> These documents are then used to enhance the care of the individual either in a home setting or in the next medical interaction. For example, one patient had to go to an emergency room in another city and presented the attending physicians with the output of the coupler; the physician called to compliment the work and tell how much it improved his ability to provide care for the patient. Moreover, we have discovered that when the prognosis and potential interventions are discussed with family members present, the beneficial involvement and awareness of these relatives of the patient increase tremendously.

These phenomena illustrate the power of shifting knowledge and information processing from the human mind to external tools. "There is something about the output of the software," the study found, "that makes a wide spectrum of concerned people become proactive" (p. 31).

As discussed above: knowledge coupling software is designed to be integrated with other elements of a reformed system of care. One of the most important of these elements is the medical record. In this regard, the study observed: "the attractiveness, acceptability, speed and efficiency of use, versatility, and power to improve care and health markedly, and many other qualities of the PKC software and its database, would, without any doubt, be greatly advanced by its integration directly into [the VA's computerized patient record system]. Based on the strong need for our veterans to receive medical care that is best practice or world class, the experience of our intervention team with both CPRS and the PKC software, the very positive findings of the present evaluation, we recommend unequivocally that the VA do this full integration into CPRS now" (p. 35). The VA never acted on that recommendation.

---

from a specialist provider should, as much as possible, be captured in the software tools. Doing so improves the tools and minimizes dependence on scarce and expensive expert specialists.

2. The MHS Study

M. Apkon et al., A Randomized Outpatient Trial of a Decision-Support Information Technology Tool, Arch Intern Med. 2005; 165:2388-2394, available at http:// archinte.ama-assn.org/cgi/reprint/165/20/2388.

This study describes a randomized controlled trial of PKC knowledge coupling software conducted at two military health system (MHS) facilities in 2002. The primary variable studied was quality of care, based on an array of process measures. Also studied were resource use, patient satisfaction and provider satisfaction. As compared to the VA study described above, this study involved a different methodology, a much larger patient population and less favorable results for the software.

We begin by summarizing the study as it is presented in the *Archives of Internal Medicine* article. We then analyze a basic conceptual flaw in the study and also examine several other elements that undermine its utility. Our central point is that the study fails to apply the basic principle, discussed in part IV.D above, knowledge coupling software, other innovations and the status quo should all be judged on how they contribute to building a total *system* of care.

Summary

Methodology. The study examined patient care using PKC Couplers with "usual care" for ambulatory patients at two military treatment facilities in Mayport, Florida and Ft. Knox, Kentucky. At these two sites, 1,902 patients participated from April to December 2002. Of these participants, 477 were excluded from the analysis for various reasons. Of the remainder, 721 patients were included in the intervention group and 704 in the control group (the two groups are referred to as the Coupler group and usual-care group, respectively). The two groups were generally similar in various respects enumerated by the study.

Patients in the Coupler group completed a Coupler "appropriate to their specific complaint or, when no condition-specific Coupler was appropriate, a generic History and Screening Coupler" (p. 2389). Thirty minutes was allocated to the process of completing the Couplers. Providers treating these patients could enter additional information before reviewing Coupler outputs outlining diagnostic or treatment options. Patients in the usual-care group had no exposure to Couplers. The initial patient encounter for both groups is referred to as the "index visit."

The study examined quality of care by comparing the Coupler and usual-care groups with respect to 24 process measures. Selected in advance of the index visits, these measures (or "opportunities for quality care") were equally divided between screening/prevention and acute/chronic disease management. The study examined the extent to which these opportunities were "fulfilled" after the index visit. Specifically:

> For each patient, the processes (or opportunities) indicated at the index visit were tabulated based on the patient's medical characteristics. Structured medical record abstraction and data from the Military Health System's electronic medical system (Composite Healthcare System) were used to determine whether each of these opportunities was satisfied ("fulfilled") within 60 days of the index visit. The primary outcome was the overall proportion of opportunities fulfilled in each study group.

To be included in the analysis, a patient had to have at least one valid "opportunity" to receive one of the 24 measured processes, meaning that if none of those processes was found to be indicated for a patient at the index visit, then the patient would be excluded. To illustrate the analysis, alcohol screening was found to be indicated for 79 patients in the Coupler group and 68 patients in the usual-care group; medical records showed that providers ordered alcohol screening for 51 patients (64.6%) in the Coupler group and 36 patients (52.9%) in the usual-care group (see the table below). "Patients were analyzed on an intention-to-treat basis" (p. 2390), apparently meaning that the study examined whether providers ordered the indicated services (as reflected in medical records), not whether follow-up occurred to ensure that patients actually received those services.

The methodology for the other dimensions of care examined by the study was as follows:

- *Resource use.* The study determined the cost of services received for 60 days after the index visit in four areas: ambulatory visits, laboratory testing, diagnostic imaging and pharmacy use. These services were identified from the electronic medical record system, and dollar values were assigned using public information as described in the study.

- *Patient and provider satisfaction.* A standard survey form was distributed to patients at their index visit. Providers were surveyed as to whether they agreed that Couplers had a positive impact in eight areas: (1) quality of care, (2) medical decision making (including impact on taking histories, conducting physical examinations, formulating diagnoses, and clinical management), (3) other benefits to patients, (4) patient satisfaction (as reported by providers), (5) patient-provider interaction, (6) time required for patient care, (7) quality of the medical knowledge base, and (8) software design and user interface.

In addition to examining the Coupler and usual-care groups, the study also examined usual-care in an "external control" clinic at a site where providers were not exposed to Couplers. This control was intended to determine whether the usual-care providers' exposure to Couplers at the two primary sites may have affected actions taken for the usual-care group. In addition, the study examined medical records of prior patients at each of the primary sites ("historical control" groups). This control was intended to account for baseline differences in quality between the study and external control clinics.

Results. With respect to the 24 quality of care measures, the study found "no significant difference in the proportion of health care opportunities fulfilled in the Coupler and usual-care groups (33.9% vs 30.7%; p = .12)." This conclusion was not altered after statistically adjusting for age, sex, military status, visit type, opportunity type, and site (p. 2391). The article provides considerable further explanation of the findings (pp. 2391-93). Table 2 in the study shows the results for the two primary sites separately and combined. The following excerpt from Table 2 shows the combined results (data are given as opportunities fulfilled/ total opportunities (percentage)):

Opportunity type	Coupler group (n = 2374)	Usual-care group (n = 2265)	P value
Screening/prevention			
Alcohol screening	51/79 (64.6)	36/68 (52.9)	.07†
Breast cancer	3/11 (27.3)	4/12 (33.3)	.43
Cervical cancer	26/95 (27.4)	22/98 (22.4)	.47
Chlamydia	22/73 (30.1)	19/64 (29.7)	.90
Colorectal cancer	4/32 (12.5)	2/58 (3.4)	.15
Depression	164/422 (38.9)	155/419 (37.0)	.58
Dietary counseling	149/493 (30.2)	108/449 (24.1)	.04
Exercise counseling	157/509 (30.8)	109/462 (23.6)	.01
Lipid	13/49 (26.5)	18/48 (37.5)	.32
Pneumococcal vaccine	1/61 (1.6)	0/72 (0.0)	.25
Smoking/advice to quit	92/209 (44.0)	101/200 (50.5)	.14
Smoking screening	40/41 (97.6)	29/33 (87.9)	.08†
Subtotal	**722/2074 (34.8)**	**603/1983 (30.4)**	**.03**

Acute/chronic			
Asthma	12/18 (66.7)	8/16 (50.0)	.57
Back pain imaging	4/4 (100.0)	2/2 (100)	NA
Back pain treatment	0/4	2/2 (100)	.05
Diabetes—ACE inhibitor	0/2	1/1 (100)	NA
Diabetes—eye examination	2/15 (13.3)	3/16 (18.8)	.75
Diabetes—hypertension	2/2 (100)	1/1 (100.)	NA
Diabetes—glycosylated hemoglobin	3/6 (50.0)	1/3 (33.3)	.48
GERD	22/138 (15.9)	19/114 (16.7)	.85
Hypertension	7/7 (100)	3/7 (42.9)	.03†
Lipid abnormalities	12/66 (18.2)	11/69 (15.9)	.81
Rhinosinusitis	2/3 (66.7)	1/1 (100)	.56
Upper respiratory tract infection	17/35 (48.6)	40/50 (80.0)	.01
Subtotal	**83/300 (27.7)**	**92/282 (32.6)**	**.26**
Total	**805/2374 (33.9)**	**695/2265 (30.7)**	**.12**

†Test of homogeneity across sites; P < .05.

With respect to resource consumption, the study found that Coupler group patients incurred higher costs for laboratory and pharmacy services than usual-care group patients, that the two groups did not differ in costs associated with ambulatory visits and radiographic evaluation, and that aggregate costs for these categories were $100 higher for the Coupler group than the usual-care group. The specific figures are shown in the following table, excerpted from Table 4 on page 2393 of the study (data are given as median (interquartile range) in dollars):

Category	Coupler group (n = 861)	Usual-care group (n = 699)	P value
Ambulatory visits	307 (153-613)	292 (146-541)	.17
Laboratory testing	43 (0-144)	31 (0-139)	.04
Diagnostic imaging	31 (0-148)	29 (0-127)	.26
Pharmacy use	203 (68-495)	164 (50-453)	.03
Total	789 (375-1654)	698 (340-1530)	.05

With respect to patient satisfaction, the study found no significant differences in any of the dimensions surveyed. With respect to provider satisfaction, the study stated the results as follows, based on surveying 8 physicians, 3 physician assistants, and 1 nurse practitioner:

> The strongest level of perceived satisfaction related to information quality: 75% agreed or strongly agreed that Couplers provides high-quality information. The strongest level of dissatisfaction related to time use, with 83% disagreeing or strongly disagreeing that Coupler use involves acceptable amounts of time. More than half of the providers also disagreed with the statements of benefits for medical decision making (70%), improved provider-patient interactions (61%), and overall benefits to patients (70%). [p. 2392]

Analysis

In both concept and execution, this study is unsound. This is apparent from an extraordinary result that the study reveals but ignores. With or without Couplers, the providers fulfilled a remarkably low proportion—only about one third—of "opportunities for quality care." Regardless of the effect of Couplers, this high rate of failure to provide quality care raises two obvious questions: to what extent did the providers fail to *identify* opportunities for quality care (a failure of decision making), and to what extent did they fail to *act on* identified opportunities (a failure of execution)?

Distinguishing between these two types of failure is essential in a study that purports to evaluate a decision support tool such as Couplers. The tool can fairly be evaluated for how well it helps identify quality opportunities (assuming the tool is used as intended), but the tool cannot fairly be evaluated for how well providers act on those opportunities, once identified. Stated differently, if the baseline reality is that providers fail to act on identified opportunities for quality, then improvement in that baseline will not result from introducing a tool whose purpose is to help identify such opportunities. This is the case no matter how successful the tool may be in accomplishing its limited purpose.

Ignoring this fundamental point, the study merely examined whether providers acted on quality opportunities (by entering orders for indicated procedures in medical records within 60 days of the index visit). On that basis, the study finds the Couplers ineffective, because the marginal difference in fulfillment rates between the Coupler and usual-care groups (33.9% vs. 30.7%; P = .12) was not statistically significant. Yet, measuring ultimate fulfillment rates does not distinguish among cases where quality opportunities were and were not identified by the Couplers, cases where quality opportunities were and were not identified by the usual-care provider, and cases where identified opportunities were and were not acted on by providers in either the Coupler group or the usual-care group.

By thus failing to distinguish between failures of decision making and failures of execution, the study failed to evaluate Couplers as a decision support tool. Beyond that, the study design and execution are full of problems. Consider the following.

- Table 2 of the study reveals a large difference in fulfillment rates between the two sites, especially for screening/prevention measures. The aggregate figures are as follows:

Opportunity type	Site 1		Site 2	
	Coupler	Usual-care	Coupler	Usual-care
Screening/Prev	21.1%	17.5%	48.3%	43.9%
Acute/chronic	23.6%	28.9%	31.1%	37.4%
Total	21.4%	19.0%	46.0%	43.1%

  Some individual measures exhibited much larger differences. For example, the Coupler/Usual-care fulfillment rates for depression screening were 13.9/10.6% for site 1 and 81.4/91.2% for site 2. These large differences between the two sites suggest that some crucial unknown variable was a primary determinant of fulfillment rates. That element further undermines any attempt to draw conclusions about the effect of Couplers.

- The study does not take into account the possibility that there might be good reason *not* to fulfill a particular quality opportunity during the 60-day measurement period. The reasonableness of a provider's actions in that regard cannot be judged in isolation from the context of the patient's complete medical needs and circumstances. A total system of care would document those needs and circumstances, and require the provider to justify decisions not to fulfill quality opportunities, using rigorous, problem-oriented medical records.

- Medical record review by trained record abstractors was apparently relied upon both to identify quality opportunities and to measure fulfillment rates. The Coupler data itself was not examined, because it was not integrated into the medical records. The reliability and consistency of this process are far from clear, given its dependence on the record-keeping practices of providers and its disconnect from the detailed documentation automatically generated by Couplers. In particular, the Coupler output is tailored to the patient's personal characteristics and the medical problem for which the Coupler is designed. These advantages of Couplers, and their effect on identification and fulfillment of quality opportunities, could not be reliably measured based on medical record review alone.

- Moreover, it is not clear that the study's measurements of opportunity fulfillment took into account that Coupler output is personalized. To illustrate, for a GERD patient who smokes, the relevant Coupler would generate advice to quit smoking, but would omit this advice for a GERD patient who does not smoke. It is not at all clear that the study took this aspect of Couplers into account when measuring the rate at which quality opportunities were fulfilled.

- According to the study, "Patients randomized to use Couplers completed the one appropriate for their specific complaint," if such a condition-specific Coupler was available. In reality, the effect of the randomization process was that many patients used a Coupler that was not appropriate for them, while other patients did not have the opportunity to use a Coupler that would have been appropriate.

- According to the study, "when no condition-specific Coupler was appropriate, a generic History and Screening Coupler" was used. In reality, providers at one of the sites (Kentucky) did not want to use the History and Screening Coupler (due to perceived liability concerns) and were permitted to use PKC's Wellness Coupler instead. Thus at the two sites, different tools were evaluated for populations to which the same tool should have been applied—a fact not disclosed in the study. It was as if half of a study cohort were permitted to use a different drug than the one under evaluation.

- Providers were not permitted to use Couplers for follow-up appointments, contrary to the manner in which Couplers should be used in practice.

- The study recites that Coupler group patients used more laboratory and pharmacy resources than usual-care group patients (no difference was found in the costs associated with ambulatory visits and radiographic evaluation). The underlying study report acknowledges: "Our analysis does not measure the clinical value and appropriateness of this resource use" (p. 74)—a statement omitted from the published article. The omitted statement defeats the negative inference about cost-effectiveness that readers would naturally draw from the published article.

- The published study characterizes provider satisfaction in largely negative terms. Yet, there are many reasons to expect that providers would not be satisfied with Couplers and the deep changes in practice they entail. Moreover, the original study includes extensive quotes from provider interviews contradicting the study's basic conclusion that Couplers are ineffective. Providers repeatedly acknowledged that Couplers informed them of relevant clinical points they might otherwise have overlooked. The provider comments included other favorable observations as well, while many of the negative comments merely reflected a basic lack of acceptance of the changes that Couplers are intended to bring about. Moreover, negative comments illustrate the core concept that an external tool like Couplers is open to feedback and organized, reproducible improvement in a way that the minds of practitioners are not.

APPENDIX B

Scientific principles that tell us why people must manage their own health care

The following reproduces the Introduction to *Your Health Care and How to Manage It*, by Lawrence L. Weed (1975).

The "scientific approach" to solving problems is a set of rules to reduce mistakes and increase benefits as we interpret our observations and the results of our actions. The rules are commonplace and easy to understand. They are not always easy to follow in complex situations such as the interactions between patients and health care providers. Review of some of the rules quickly reveals why the patients themselves must become actively involved; it is the only way we shall control the overuse and misuse of drugs and procedures and the rising costs in the medical care system.

Variables:

The more variables you know and consider in a situation, the wiser you can be in that situation. The more continuous the observation of the variables, the smoother the necessary adjustments can be.

In maintaining health, in chronic disease, and in the events that lead to acute illness, the patients themselves know and control more of the relevant variables than anyone else. Patients live with the variables all the time. When the values of those variables change (when the situation changes), they can be the first to know.

Physicians often know only a few of the variables and usually have direct control over none. Physicians and other medical personnel see a fragment of the total during a fragment of the time.

Examples:

1. Managing Variables in a Chronic Disease
    In a diabetic in which we use the blood sugar level as a goal and index of control, the following variables are some that are known to affect it:

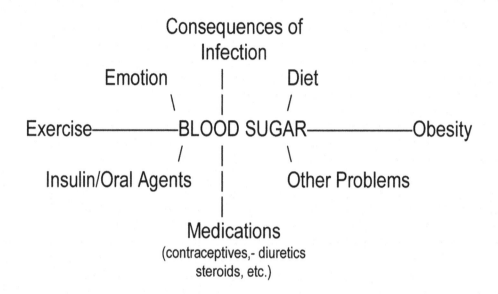

2. Understanding and managing variables that predispose to acute disease:

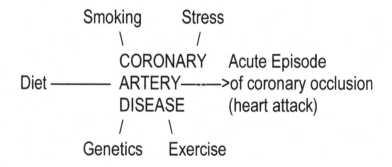

The patient is aware of and has control over more of the above variables than anyone else. The physician goes to medical school and tries to learn textbook averages about many diseases. The patient knows many things that the disease does to him; the facts are his with no formal education at all.

Therefore:

Responsibility for health care rests in the patient's hands because that is where the knowledge of and control of the variables lie. To meet this responsibility, the patient needs:

1. The conviction that it is his responsibility to look at the variables and to act upon them. Previous data on similar patients can give some guidance, but only his own exact past data can tell him what adjustments must be made. This has to be so because no two people are exactly the same combination of variables.

2. The correct tools and guidance to interpret and act upon the variables wisely.

3. Above all the patient needs the responsibility itself; otherwise a dependency state is created, self-respect is lost, motivation diminishes, and the patient withdraws—leaving the situation to professional providers who cannot control or even know about many of the variables.

————

Variables and Records:

Keeping track of variables over time and examining for crucial inter-relationships are beyond the capacity of the unaided human mind. Records are necessary.

Patients can capitalize upon their awareness of and continuous exposure to most of the variables by learning to keep and read their own records, including graphs and flowsheets. They can discern their own unique patterns of response and be the first to see what works and what does not work. The data can protect them from their own unfounded notions and from the misconceptions and generalizations of those who treat them.

Furthermore, they will not charge for keeping the record, they will not run out of storage room, there will be one medical librarian for each record in the country, and accessibility/retrieval problems as the patient moves around should be minimal. Patients will not have to repeat their story and explain what pills and tests they have had every time they see a new medical person. They will not always have to be wondering whether the physician or nurse knows all he should as he starts new and serious treatments.

Patients and society will not have to pay the bill for all the inefficiencies that result from the redundancies and poor communication in the medical profession.

Providers specialize and a single patient is treated by more than one specialist. Each specialist keeps a separate record for each patient, and each patient is unaware of that record's contents; therefore, crucial information is not readily available when it is needed. When institutions run out of storage space and money for proper record maintenance, the patient pays for the confusion and lack of availability of needed information.

When patients visit the office of a specialist or when they are admitted to a hospital, including the academic medical centers, it is not the custom to simply add the necessary new information and plans to a single, cumulative account of the individual's health status. Much of the information from physician's offices and personal memories is not even available, let alone organized in a form common to all. Rather, patients are "worked-up" from scratch— repeatedly, and this process takes hours of extra time; providers often skip crucial information from past records as a result. There is no good system whereby efforts are cumulative and coordinated; the result is that the right hand does not know what the left hand is doing. Some physicians try to solve the problem by extreme dedication and overwork, but they frequently end up disillusioned and dissatisfied. This is particularly true of house officers who may admit as many as five patients in one evening, each with a few words scribbled on a prescription blank from the person who sent them in. Since providers do not simply add to a single, complete, organized, cumulative record, the house officer stays up all night and, even then, does not get the job done properly. Furthermore, there is a tradition in doctor training and practice to do your "night on" alone no matter what the load. Support from second and third back-up call systems is not used so that patients can be guaranteed adequate attention. The patient admitted alone on one night with a thoughtful superior doctor is in very different circumstances from the one admitted with five other patients on the same night when all are under the care of a less skilled physician. Patients and families of patients must be aware of these realities so that they can begin to mobilize cumulative accounts -of their own situation and actively help the providers bring the information under control.

Also, because coordination is so bad, logic so poorly preserved in the written record, and medical personnel rely so much on -fallible human memories for information on patients and medical knowledge, intelligent analysis of medical action on populations of patients is all but impossible on a routine basis. Many of our mistakes go undetected. Occasionally, a disease like Legionnaires' disease will erupt and the government will spend thousands of dollars trying to piece together past actions from scattered, disorganized, and illegible records which were never checked for quality in the first place. Or occasionally an academic person will study a subject like antibiotic use and find, as they recently published in an article from Duke University, that 64% of the time the wrong antibiotic is given or the wrong dose is used. How much worse does medicine have to get before the medical establishment realizes and admits that there is something wrong with this disorganized, memory-based, uncoordinated, inefficient system for communication and problem solving?

Therefore:

The patient must have a copy of his own record. He must be involved with organizing and recording the variables so that the course of his own data on disease and treatment will slowly reveal to him what the best care for him should be. Crippling dependency states in patients will be fewer. Needless repetition of expensive and dangerous medical activities will be controlled.

It is true that there are those who live to a ripe, old age, are rarely sick, have handled what medical problems they have with natural body defenses and no medical records. Compulsive thinking about health and medical record keeping could do more harm to them than good. We can certainly let them continue in the successful medical approaches they have worked out for themselves. But for those who are not always healthy and have not found personal approaches that work for them and who continuously turn to the medical profession for guidance, and upon whom actions are taken and records kept (good and bad), we are merely saying that these individuals must get involved, must understand the actions and records, and must study the results of the interventions. Otherwise, they could be victims of some of the bad effects that disorganized medical activity can generate.

Relationships Among Variables:

Scientists record and observe the course of variables to look for trends and associations among them. To separate coincidence from cause and effect, they observe many times and use mathematical *techniques to analyze. Some relationships are simple to see; every time the temperature gets low the water freezes; others are more subtle. Scientists hypothesize and manipulate variables to bring out relationships, but they try to change one at a time so they will know what is causing what. They do not draw conclusions beyond what the data will support.*

In medicine, particularly in chronic disease, the patient continually lives with the variables and knows better than anyone else when many, not just one, are changing. He knows that conclusions about what is causing what should be made with great caution. At the present time patients have little access to the data and the physician's thought processes. In their ignorance of these facts and with unfounded expectations for an "instant cure," they develop exaggerated ideas of the physician's power and demand diagnostic con-clusions at times when none are possible. In an honest medical setting, none are possible much more than half the time. Patients need to be taught a tolerance of ambiguity; it can be tolerated when they have access to the data and the physician's logic concerning their problems.

Physicians and other medical providers are away from the patients and the variables most of the time. They write an order to change one variable like an ijisulin4ose and assume the others to be constant (which they rarely are). It is very common for the very same physicians who fail to get enough data or to organize the variables at the outset to also be the ones who introduce too many new, uncontrolled variables (excessive ordering of laboratory tests, procedures, and drugs). Furthermore they analyze and interpret the results either inadequately or sometimes not at all; they needlessly change too many variables at once, and draw conclusions from uncontrolled situations and from numbers of cases that are not statistically significant. The pressure from uninformed patients for diagnosis and predictions increases these tendencies among providers.

Even when physicians change just one variable in the analysis of one problem, they may completely ignore the effects of that change on the other problems. Furthermore, many physicians try to deal with all this complexity in their heads—without good records, without carefully constructed flowsheets and graphs; there is no organization of data to help them avoid mistakes, and without such organized data, they may fail to recognize their own mistakes. Their confidence goes on undisturbed.

Therefore:

Patients must know what providers are thinking, what they are trying to do or demonstrate, what the variables are so that they can protect the provider and themselves from invalid conclusions. Good science and good medicine are not just accurate data, not just a lot of data, and not just a brilliant analysis of some of the data. They are all three, and it takes a cooperative approach with adequate tools to achieve all three. Records cannot do it alone, providers cannot do it alone, patients cannot do it alone, and guidance tools cannot do it all alone.

They must be coupled into a smoothly working unit. It is not "The Record," "My Doctor," "That Computer" — it is the right combination to identify and solve the problem.

The right combination is very difficult to achieve consistently. That is why massive expenditures on specialized parts of the body do not achieve massive improvements in mortality and morbidity statistics. Matters could get worse because even the marvelous balancing mechanisms of nature that have evolved over millions of years cannot keep up with the uncontrolled interventions of increasing numbers of people who make their living manipulating variables in the general population, all~ in the name of "medical care."

The medical schools are the worst offenders. They teach and examine for facts out of all proportion to teaching and examining for the capacity to collect and organize data effectively, control variables, and draw conclusions rigorously. The transmission of the medical school faculty's scientific facts often overwhelms — even precludes — the transmission of scientific behavior to students. The failures in medical education are, in their own way, every bit as bad as the failures in grade school education that are now so widely discussed. Discipline and follow through on medical actions are largely absent in much of medical practice today. The simple principles taught in the sixth grade general science courses are violated day after day in patient care. Patients must understand that even if medical schools were to change tomorrow (and they will not), it would be years before that change would help them.

THE SCIENTIFIC PRINCIPLES ARE SIMPLE, AND YOU CAN APPLY THEM TO YOURSELF IMMEDIATELY IN YOUR OWN THINKING ABOUT YOUR OWN MEDICAL CARE. STOP EXPECTING THE "IMPOSSIBLE" FROM THE MEDICAL PROFESSION AND START DOING THE "POSSIBLE" FOR YOURSELF.

Variables From Mind and Body:

Variables in real problems do not follow the boundaries of academic disciplines. Identifying as many relevant variables as possible should precede the analysis and manipulation of the few variables that are easily seen and understood by the specialist.

In health and disease there is no boundary line between ~the mind and the body. The patients naturally see the flow from one to the other. It is common to hear them say: "She comes home with tummy aches when she has that teacher." "He's continually fighting with his boss; he better watch his blood pressure." "The in-laws hadn't been there two days when she had a migraine and an asthmatic attack." –

Physicians divide themselves into psychiatric services, medical services, surgical services, etc. The flow of mind-body relationships is often not perceived across their man-made boundaries. The work-up for the back pain on the orthopedic service looks completely different from the work-up for the back pain on the psychiatric service. .

You are in the best position to keep data that could reveal true cause and effect-relationships among mental and physical events. Physicians and other providers may be either paternalistic and draw conclusions and make judgments on only a few of the variables and without consultation with you, the patient; or they may act too hastily on undocumented, verbal, anecdotal notions of patients about cause and effect.

Therefore:

Providers must encourage the patient to keep his own data; the provider must share all the data he has and must review his interpretations with the patient so that the patient in turn can critically review what is being done and accept the obligation of changing it if he does not understand or agree. And, if the providers do not encourage or offer to share and review, then patients must demand the information.

A goal should be to let the data speak to both the~ patient and the provider and have record keeping tools to accomplish that.

We do not need compulsive documentation of the normal, daily interactions, but when troubles and problems appear, we must not improvise hasty solutions from the patient's or doctor's memory.

———

Motivation Versus Knowledge:
Really wanting to know and taking the time to find out are what lead to scientific advances and a body of knowledge and understanding.

In theft own health problems, people are naturally motivated to ask questions and seek answers. They can also solve problems if they are given the proper tools and enough time, even if their knowledge is deficient at the outset. Knowledge help is found all over once you start to look for it—in public libraries, the latest edition of the Encyclopedia Britannica, pamphlets of all sorts from numerous agencies and many departments of the federal government. The individual's own medical record is the basic tool he needs to organize and pursue the problems and the information related to them.

PHYSICIANS AND OTHER PROVIDERS ARE NOT NATURALLY MOTIVATED TO ASK QUESTIONS AND STATE PROBLEMS FROM THE PATIENT'S POINT OF VIEW. THEY CONTINUALLY SEE THINGS IN TERMS OF THE WAY THEY WERE TRAINED AND - THE SPECIALTY THEY ENTERED. This gives them the skill and drive necessary to solve a problem in their area once it is presented, but it does not lead them to naturally organize and review all the problems and set priorities from the patient's point of view.

Therefore:

Patients must be educated in the use of tools such as the problem-oriented record and computerized POMR so that there is some concrete instrument for expressing and capitalizing upon their own motivation. If the patients are not motivated enough to use the tools effectively, then we should get over the illusion that those same patients are accomplishing much with twenty minute visits to providers or that they are complying very precisely with directions from those providers, except in those instances where a normally healthy individual gets specialized care for a self-limited problem from the appropriate specialist, e.g. a broken leg.

———

The Power Of The Right Tools:
Tools extend our muscles, our senses, our memories, and our analytical capacities. Extending our muscles and our senses with automobiles, power tools, telescopes, etc. are commonplace. Extending our basically chemical and electronic minds with electronic computers is becoming more commonplace.

For patients who, up until now, have had little exposure in school or elsewhere to the use of the medical record as a powerful tool in their own health care, the particular form of this tool will be of little consequence so long as it is clear to them and usable by them. A computerized problem-oriented record will not be any newer or more confusing to them than traditional paper records since they never had either record in the past.

Physicians, nurses, and other providers have been trained with a whole set of habits and notions about medical records and their availability to patients. It is difficult for some of them to switch to electronic tools that provide specific guidance for solving problems within the context of patients' other problems. Some not only do not want to switch to an~ electronic record system, they still do not recognize that the record should be a tool the patient's use as much as a tool for their own use.

Therefore:

In health care, patients and very inexpensive paramedical people who are already a permanent part of a community must-be taught to use the problem solving guidance in their own records and eventually in computers. After all, rescue squads with remarkable skill in heart and lung disease have been developed all over the country, and people with only a high school education or less have been taught to do sophisticated medical work. Surely we all can learn to deal with many of the less life-threatening disorders such as sore throats and body aches if we have our records and the right guidance tools. Expensively trained medical professionals should be reserved for specialized tasks that we cannot master and cannot do for ourselves. They also should be used to build the guidance in the tools and to monitor occasionally our records and behaviors to make sure that we are behaving in a disciplined and reliable manner.

———

Uniqueness:

Multiple variables, constantly changing, continuously create unique combinations. If one hundred different people were each to drive from New York to Los Angeles, we could not predict accurately their exact routes. A road map of the United States shows all the major towns and an enormous number of highways connecting them. The map facilitates travel—the unique requirements of the traveler determine which of the many paths is chosen.

Every patient is a unique traveler through the medical landscape. There are no two patients—even with the same disease—who have the same manifestations, the same course, and the same qualitative and quantitative constellation of accompanying problems. Nor do they have the same goals and same resources to reach those goals. But, just as the same map can be given to and used by many travelers, so the best medical options can be given to each person as he and the provider slowly work their way, step by step, through a medical or social problem.

Determining the best regimen for an individual in chronic disease and the best program for prevention for what appears to be just acute, episodic disease (e.g., the perforated ulcer) is always a matter of research because of the uniqueness of individuals.

Patterns of Uniqueness: Although a patient is/1 ~ unique, his unique patterns of illness and response to treatment tend to repeat themselves in recurrences of a given disease and even in different diseases. In other words, how a patient gets sick is more related to his constitutional background and habits than to the outside agent causing his illness. Expose a group of people to the same amount of virus or bacterial agent or a simple ankle injury and notice the extremely broad spectrum of responses. The patient has only his problem or problems to be concerned with and years to master his responsibilities.

Physicians and other medical providers and scientists have organized medical knowledge in terms of diseases, emphasizing those manifestations of the disease that are common to the largest number of people with the disease. In medical care review they divide people up into groups of people with a given disease and look for common findings and treatments in judging the care of a disease. When medical plans and procedures are ordered, they are frequently done on the basis of this medical knowledge in medical textbooks. Frequently, the medical knowledge about the unique patient kept in the individual patient record is ignored in favor of textbook averages. Medical care is too often not tailored to an individual's unique needs as defined by his previously recorded, unique patterns.

Therefore:

The patient must understand his uniqueness if he is to understand why he must have a primary role in his own care and if he is to control his unrealistic expectations. The patient must understand that, because he is unique, the results of any medical intervention cannot be predicted with absolute confidence. Follow-through and adjustments are everything as the data unfold. The patient, it is true, may not do his part, but at least we can get him over the illusion that anyone can do it for him. For many aspects of management, a physician's partially-recalled knowledge cannot possibly compete with a patient's organized knowledge of himself. Our job is to give the patient the tools and responsibility to organize the knowledge and slowly learn to integrate it. This can be done with modern guidance tools.

The patient must be made aware of the above principle and its implications for his responsibility in his own care. He must first think through the past and then tell those helping him what he thinks the future course will be on the basis of his detailed knowledge of his past reactions and behaviors. Uninformed providers now discover things through painful experiences and unnecessary trial and error. They also draw the wrong conclusions from the limited, parochial variables they so painstakingly analyze. Specialization and limiting the patient's role suppress whole series of variables that profoundly affect outcomes.

———

Time and Achievement:

Most scientists seek a certain level of achievement, and they adjust the time spent and the number of tasks attempted accordingly. To the' extent that a non-fiction writer misjudges his own work, the editor of the journal is expected to judge it further, and if it is not up to a certain standard, it is sent back for further work or further drafts. The amount of time the investigator has spent or the number of other things he is working on count for nothing in the evaluation of the work.

Among people both sick and well, there are no two who will take the same time to master their responsibilities in their own health care. Unfortunately, in all of their education, they have been treated as if people are equal and should arrive at the same standards in the same time. They took the same number of courses over the same number of school years. When the results were different, instead of saying "the data show us our system is wrong" (some require more time than others to do things correctly), we said "some are better or worse than others," gave grades and prizes, punishment and disgrace and drove them all on to the next step leaving a trail of tasks done poorly.

Physicians and other providers often make time the constant and achievement the variable with patients. They try to do everything for the patient themselves and even keep all the records to themselves and instruct the patients hurriedly over a series of timed appointments. They do not have the time or money to give the necessary time to those who need it; on the other hand, they also have patients who return for repeated office visits that are unnecessary because those patients understood their situation at the first visit and can manage their own affairs. In such medical practices the patient is not only being denied his essential role as an informed participant. in his care, he is also being denied the basis to form an accurate judgment about the quality of health care he is purchasing.

Therefore:

Responsibility for quality must, in large part, rest with the patient. A patient can make time the variable in his own health care and stick to something until it is mastered, once he is given the responsibility to do so—like working out the right insulin dosage. A provider must audit until the necessary result is achieved and must avoid overinvolvement when he is no longer needed.

The Art of Medicine:
Compassion and Scientific Principles

Compassion and Responsibility:

The most compassionate thing to do in the long run is to do things right. For all the common sense reasons and scientific reasons given above, each individual has to do much for himself if the right things are ever to be done. The most effective way to be responsible to others is first of all to be responsible for ourselves and not be a burden to others. We can show our compassion for others by helping them be independent. Compassion that creates dependency states in others is a misguided compassion that demoralizes and destroys.

The Art of Medicine:

Finally you may ask where - does the art of medicine fit in? Surely no system will make one kind, thoughtful, or sympathetic: to care deeply about the plight of others is a quality not dispensed in manuals of any type. But to say that the art of medicine is not dependent on a great - deal of discipline and order is to miss perhaps the true understanding of what underlies art in any form. The physician as well as the musician and poet should read the following words of Stravinsky and at least recognize the possibility that they also apply to him:

> A mode of composition that does not assign itself limits becomes pure fantasy. The effect it produces may accidentally amuse, but is not capable of being repeated. The creator's function is to sift the elements he receives, for human activity must impose limits upon itself. The more art is controlled, limited, worked over, the more it is free.

> As for myself, I experience a sort of terror when, at the moment of setting to work and finding myself before the infinitude of possibilities that present themselves, I have the feeling that everything is permissible to me. If everything is permissible to me, the best and the worst; if nothing offers me any resistance, then any effort is inconceivable, and I cannot use anything as a basis, and consequently, every undertaking becomes futile.

> What delivers me from the anguish into which an unrestricted freedom plunges me is the fact that I am always able to turn immediately to the concrete things that are here in question. I have no use for a theoretic freedom. Let me have something finite, definite—matter that can lend itself to my operation only insofar as it is commensurate with

my possibilities. And such matter presents itself to me together with its limitations. I must in turn impose mine upon it. So here we are, whether we like it or not, in the realm of necessity. And yet which of us has ever heard talk of art as other than a realm of freedom? This sort of heresy is uniformly widespread because it is imagined that art is outside the bounds of ordinary activity. Well, in art as in everything else, one can build only upon a resisting foundation: whatever constantly gives way to pressure constantly renders movement impossible.

My freedom thus consists in my moving about within the narrow frame that I have assigned myself for each one of my undertakings.

Authors' Background and Acknowledgements

Lawrence L. Weed, MD, has held positions in a number of academic and health care institutions. Aspects of his experience that led to the work described in this book are briefly discussed at note 158 above and in "Idols of the Mind," especially pp. 4-6, at http://www.ihi.org/ihi/Files/Forum/2006/Handouts/P4_LWeed_Idols_of_the_Mind_IIb.pdf. Further background on LLW is available from "The Computer Will See You Now," *The Economist*, Dec. 8, 2005, at http://www.economist.com/node/5269189. He can be reached at ll.weed@comcast.net.

Lincoln Weed, JD, LLW's son, practiced employee benefits law in Washington, D.C. for 26 years. In 2009, he joined a consulting firm, Axiom Resource Management, Inc., where he specializes in health information privacy. His experience as an employee benefits lawyer included work on health benefits. This intersection with LLW's work in medicine led to co-authoring two articles with LLW, published in 1994 and 1999 (cited in note 38 and at the end of note 2). He can be reached at ldweed424@gmail.com.

* * *

This book reflects the work of many people over many years. In particular, the authors wish to acknowledge contributions of the following. Harold Cross, MD began working with LLW more than 50 years ago on implementing the concepts of the problem-oriented medical record. His work was indispensable to everything that followed. The authors' son/brother Chris Weed, whose writings are cited repeatedly in this book, has been integral to creation of knowledge coupling software and the electronic problem-oriented medical record over the past 30 years. His deep understanding of both philosophical and technical issues has been important to those working in software development and medical content development, and it informs every page of this book.

Finally, and above all, Laura Brooks Weed, MD (1922-1997), for more than four decades contributed enormously to the work described in this book. As a highly qualified and experienced physician, she was a source of invaluable insight and advice on many levels (including building much of the initial medical content for knowledge coupling software). In addition to her professional roles, she was a tower of strength and support to her family and everyone who knew her.

Made in the USA
Columbia, SC
29 March 2018